SpringerBriefs in Social Work

More information about this series at http://www.springer.com/series/13578

Lisa Schelbe · Jennifer M. Geiger

Intergenerational Transmission of Child Maltreatment

Springer

Lisa Schelbe
College of Social Work
Florida State University
Tallahassee, FL
USA

Jennifer M. Geiger
Jane Addams College of Social Work
University of Illinois at Chicago
Chicago, IL
USA

ISSN 2195-3104 ISSN 2195-3112 (electronic)
SpringerBriefs in Social Work
ISBN 978-3-319-43822-1 ISBN 978-3-319-43824-5 (eBook)
DOI 10.1007/978-3-319-43824-5

Library of Congress Control Number: 2016955066

Printed on acid-free paper

This Springer imprint is published by Springer Nature
The registered company is Springer International Publishing AG
The registered company address is: Gewerbestrasse 11, 6330 Cham, Switzerland

This book is dedicated to our partners, Chris Schoborg and Mike Geiger, and to the parents, practitioners, and researchers who work tirelessly to prevent child maltreatment.

Preface

Our interest in the intergenerational transmission of child maltreatment (ITCM) originated from our work with youth aging out of foster care. We saw firsthand how youth aging out who were parents often struggled to overcome obstacles they faced. All were striving to provide a better life for their children, but perhaps did not have the resources or support that we often take for granted as parents. We studied the experiences of youth aging out and increasingly became convinced that a potential opportunity to prevent future maltreatment was to target youth in and aging out of the foster care system. It started with our article in the *Journal of Public Child Welfare,* published in 2014 that outlined existing research and policies and the need to focus on pregnant and parenting youth in and aging out of foster care in an effort to prevent ITCM (Geiger and Schelbe 2014). We realized through our work with youth aging out how important and prevalent the experience of parenting was for youth aging out and sought ways to better understand ITCM. Neither of us has worked on empirical studies examining ITCM, yet we understand that ITCM plays a role in our work with youth aging out. Accordingly, we started our investigation of ITCM among various populations, including youth aging out in *Advances in Child Abuse Prevention Knowledge*, edited by Deb Daro, Anne Cohn Donnelly, Lee Ann Huang, and Byron Powell in 2015. We have begun to investigate the parenting attitudes of youth aging out and how they might fare as parents in the future (Geiger and Schelbe under review) and what the experiences of parents aging out are given the myriad of challenges they face in their daily life. This SpringBrief started after Jennifer Hadley at Springer read an abstract in the program of the 2014 National Conference on Child Abuse and Neglect and reached out to Lisa to gauge her interest in writing a Spring Brief on ITCM. We pursued the opportunity with the hope that this knowledge can inform future research, programs, and policies related to prevention and intervention development with parents and families.

It is our hope that this book can be a resource to students, practitioners, and researchers studying and working in the child maltreatment field. Despite decades of research and interventions, child maltreatment and its etiology remain a very complex and complicated phenomenon. This book synthesizes what is known about ITCM to guide those who are developing interventions and conducting child maltreatment prevention research. We aimed to comprehensively review what is known about ITCM, critique the current literature, and offer direction for future research and interventions. The book is based on the premise that to effectively prevent child maltreatment, understanding the nature of ITCM is of utmost importance.

Tallahassee, FL, USA Lisa Schelbe
Chicago, IL, USA Jennifer M. Geiger

Acknowledgments

Thanks to our friends and colleagues at Florida State University, Arizona State University, the University of Illinois at Chicago, and the University of Pittsburgh who supported our writing this book early in our careers. We appreciate how you served as sounding boards as we developed our tables and figures, reorganized the chapters, and processed our work.

We would like to thank the Doris Duke Charitable Foundation and the Doris Duke Fellowship for the Promotion of Child Well-being. While the book was not funded directly through the foundation, our collaboration is a direct product of our receiving Doris Duke Fellowships for the Promotion of Child Well-being. The annual meeting and other events throughout the year sponsored by the fellowship provided the foundation of our collaborative work. The Doris Duke Fellowship also provided additional training and the opportunity to be part of a network of scholars committed to preventing child abuse and neglect. Thanks to Lee Ann Huang for her tireless behind-the-scenes work that made these in-person meetings and trainings meaningful and successful. The chapters of this book are filled with references to work of Doris Duke Fellows and their mentors, as well as from many of the scholars who have spoken at Doris Duke Fellowship meetings and provided trainings and webinars. We would like to thank our fellow Doris Duke Fellows for their work and the discussions we have had over the years that have helped further our thinking about ITCM and the prevention of child maltreatment. Special thanks to Dr. Deb Daro, who makes the Doris Duke Fellowship for the Promotion of Child Well-being all that it is. Thank you all for your support over the years, and specifically your encouragement of this project. We appreciate your feedback on our prospectus.

Thanks to our families who were patient and supportive as we spent time writing this book. Your support and reassurance made this possible.

Special thanks from Lisa: I am so fortunate to have a loving supportive family. Alithea and Keven, thank you for never complaining when I needed quiet time and had to write in the evening. Jane and Kate, thank you for checking in with emoji filled texts and being my biggest cheerleaders. Mom and Dad, thank you for your ongoing support. Chris, thank you for taking care of everything and being the backbone of the home while I worked on this book. Your never-ending belief in me fueled me on the days I felt in over my head. Thank you.

Special thanks from Jen: Thank you to my amazing partner Mike for encouraging me to pursue every opportunity and for giving me the space and time to do this. I especially appreciate what an amazing father you are to our kids and how you keep our lives full of love, imagination, fun, knowledge, and exploration. You have always supported me and even pretended to be interested in the things I study and write about.

Contents

Abbreviations

ACYF	Administration for Children, Youth, and Families
ADHD	Attention Deficit Hyperactivity Disorder
CDC	Centers for Disease Control and Prevention
CSSP	Center for the Study on Social Policy
EBP	Evidence-Based Practice
IOM	Institute of Medicine
ITCM	Intergenerational Transmission of Child Maltreatment
LBGTQ	Lesbian, Gay, Bisexual, Transgender, and Queer
SSNR	Safe, Stable and Nurturing Relationships
US DHHS	United States Department of Health and Human Services
WHO	World Health Organization

Chapter 1
What Is Intergenerational Transmission of Child Maltreatment?

1.1 Intergenerational Transmission of Child Maltreatment

Intergenerational transmission of child maltreatment (ITCM) occurs when a person who was maltreated as a child maltreats his or her own children. It is a widely held belief that (1) people who abuse or neglect a child were likely abused or neglected themselves as children and that (2) children who experience abuse and neglect grow up and are more likely to abuse and neglect their own children. Scholars have pointed out that professionals also hold this belief as well despite limited empirical evidence (e.g., Garbarino and Gilliam 1980; Widom 1989a). Indeed, the concept of ITCM appears throughout the literature on child abuse and neglect.

The concept of ITCM is deceptively simple, yet before embracing it completely, we should look more closely at the theory and the research behind it. While ITCM is an appealing intuitive idea, the empirical evidence supporting it is mixed (Ertem et al. 2000; Garbarino and Gilliam 1980; Thornberry et al. 2012, Widom 1989a). A parent's history of child maltreatment is neither the only prerequisite nor a cause of future child maltreatment (Dixon et al. 2009). Studies have found a greater likelihood of parents maltreating their children if they were maltreated themselves as children (e.g., Egeland et al. 1988; Kim 2009; Widom 1989a). However, research consistently finds that the majority of people who experience child maltreatment do not go on to abuse and neglect their own children (e.g., Kaufman and Zigler 1987; Pears and Capaldi 2001; Sidebotham et al. 2006; Widom and Wilson 2015). Likewise, among adults who maltreat their children, the majority did not experience maltreatment in their own childhood (Widom 1989c). In this book, we will present the research and theoretical underpinnings of ITCM as well as the implications for future research and interventions.

L. Schelbe and J.M. Geiger, *Intergenerational Transmission of Child Maltreatment*, SpringerBriefs in Social Work,
DOI 10.1007/978-3-319-43824-5_1

1.1.1 Definition of Intergenerational Transmission of Child Maltreatment

We will first start with a definition of intergenerational transmission of child maltreatment by breaking down some of the elements of the phrase.[1] We can start at the end of the phrase first. *Child maltreatment* includes various forms of neglect and abuse of a child, or a person under the age of 18.[2] *Child neglect* at its most basic level is a parent or caregiver's failure to meet a child's basic needs such as food, clothing, shelter, security, and hygiene. A parent or caregiver may also neglect a child by providing inadequate supervision that places a child at risk. For example, a parent who is intoxicated and passed out may not prevent a hungry toddler from leaving the home and walking outside alone without shoes or a clean diaper. *Child abuse* is purposeful, specific, and repeated mistreatment from a parent or caregiver. Abuse has various forms: physical, emotional, and sexual. *Physical abuse* is non-accidental injuries inflicted upon a child and includes behaviors that may result in a child having bruises, burns, lacerations, broken bones, head injuries, and internal injuries. *Emotional abuse*, sometimes referred to as psychological abuse, broadly defined, is not creating a positive healthy atmosphere for a child. Parents or caregivers emotionally abuse a child when they repeatedly belittle, humiliate, reject, isolate, terrorize, ignore, or destroy the self-worth and esteem of a child. *Sexual abuse* includes any sexual contact and activities between a parent or caregiver and a child. While we have just presented maltreatment as distinct types of abuse and neglect, it is important to note that there is substantial overlap and high rates of co-occurrence. In the next section of the chapter, we will delve into more

---

[1]Different researchers use the term cycle of violence, which is also used as a term for intergenerational transmission of violence to mean different things. Heyman and Slep (2002) explain this well: "Further, what exactly is meant by the cycle of violence? As noted by Heyman and Ezzell (in press), different researchers use the term to mean different things, leaving at least 10 relations sharing the same moniker: (a) child victimization and/or exposure to interparental violence lead to violent criminal behavior in adolescence and/or adulthood…; child maltreatment victimization leads to (b) child maltreatment perpetration in adulthood, (c) partner abuse perpetration in adulthood, or (d) partner abuse victimization in adulthood; child exposure to interparental violence leads to (e) child maltreatment perpetration in adulthood, (f) partner abuse perpetration in adulthood, or (g) partner abuse victimization in adulthood; and child victimization and exposure to interparental violence lead to (h) child maltreatment perpetration in adulthood, (i) partner abuse perpetration in adulthood, (j) partner abuse victimization in adulthood. Despite substantial methodological problems (cf. Widom 1989a, b, c), there is weak but consistent support for the first seven hypotheses (Heyman and Ezzell, in press). The final three hypotheses lack any published empirical test" (p. 864).

[2]The Child Abuse Prevention and Treatment Act (2010) (Public Law 111–320) provides the minimum definition of child maltreatment: "the term 'child abuse and neglect' means, at a minimum, any recent act or failure to act on the part of a parent or caretaker, which results in death, serious physical or emotional harm, sexual abuse or exploitation, or an act or failure to act which presents an imminent risk of serious harm." This definition provides the basis for all states to develop laws for child maltreatment, yet legal definitions differ among the states.

background about the types of maltreatment and consequences, but right now we simply want to provide basic definitions.

To break down the concepts of *intergenerational* and *transmission*, we present Joe Q. Public and his family. When Joe was a child, his mother treated him in a certain way. When Joe had children of his own, he treated his children the same way that he had been treated. Following the same pattern, his children may grow up and treat their children in the same way that their grandmother treated their father. The way the parents in Joe's family treated their children or their behavior—in this book we will be focused on child maltreatment—happened across generations with one generation after another passing along the tradition. The mechanism of the passing along between generations—the transmission—is not fully understood, although there are several theoretical frameworks, which we will discuss in Chap. 2, which are often used to explain the phenomenon. In some ways we can conceptualize the intergenerational transmission of child maltreatment as simply a family tradition. It is important to recognize, however, that a family tradition of maltreatment is likely to be deeply imbedded in cultural and social norms and influenced by a myriad of factors.

Combining the elements we have just defined, intergenerational transmission of child maltreatment (ITCM) occurs when a child is abused or neglected by a parent or caregiver and then grows up to abuse and neglect her or his children. Arguably, this is not the entire story, as research shows: (1) the majority of people who were maltreated as children do not grow up and abuse and neglect their children (e.g., Kaufman and Zigler 1987; Pears and Capaldi 2001; Sidebotham et al. 2006; Widom and Wilson 2015) and (2) there people who were not maltreated as children who grow up and abuse and neglect their children (e.g., Dixon et al. 2009). ITCM is sometimes spoken of deterministically, however, the reality is there is more than only one risk factor for perpetrating child maltreatment in the future. As we will discuss in Chaps. 4 and 5, there are clearly protective factors and risk factors outside of a parent having a history of being maltreated.

While we have just presented ITCM in a straight forward manner, albeit with the caveat that most people do not continue a cycle of violence in their family, it is also important to describe another closely related phenomenon—the intergenerational continuity of child maltreatment. There are people who experienced maltreatment as children who have children who are abused or neglected by someone other than the parent with the history of maltreatment. This *continuity* of maltreatment is closely related to the *transmission* of maltreatment yet differs because with *continuity* the person who is perpetrating the maltreatment is not necessarily the parent who experienced maltreatment (Berlin et al. 2011; Valentino et al. 2012). Thus, instances where there is transmission of child maltreatment is a subgroup of continuity. However, it is worthwhile to note that some studies do not differentiate between the transmission and continuity of child maltreatment. For example, Marshall and colleagues (2011) explain "Intergenerational transmission of child maltreatment refers to the continuity of child maltreatment across generations" (p. 1024).

For the purpose of this book, we are concerned with the occurrence of child maltreatment across subsequent generations. Thus, with this definition of ITCM, we include studies that are arguably examining the continuity of child maltreatment (e.g., the perpetrator of the child maltreatment is unknown, or a parent who experienced the child maltreatment was not the perpetrator of child maltreatment that his/her child experienced) rather than a narrow focus that only considers the transmission where the parent who was maltreated as a child goes onto maltreat her/his child.

1.1.2 Intergenerational Transmission of Child Maltreatment and the Cycle of Violence

Before we explore child maltreatment more thoroughly, it is important to situate ITCM within the larger corpus of literature on the cycle of violence. The cycle of violence hypothesis posits that children who are maltreated are at increased risk for engaging in violence when they grow up (see Fig. 1.1). ITCM is just one element of research that examines violent behaviors of those who were maltreated as children. Studies have also examined other outcomes such as delinquent behaviors (Hubbard and Pratt 2002; Lansford et al. 2007; Schwartz et al. 1994; Smith et al. 2005; Smith and Thornberry 1995; Stouthamer-Loeber et al. 2001; Widom 1998), violent crimes (Maxfield and Widom 1996; Rivera and Widom 1990; Widom 1998, 1989b), and intimate partner violence (McKinney et al. 2009; Renner and Slack 2006; White and Widom 2003; Widom et al. 2014).

The focus of this book is specifically on child maltreatment. Delinquency, violent crime (other than that which is child maltreatment) and intimate partner violence (other than how it connects to child maltreatment) are beyond the scope of this book. This is not to say that the other topics are not important; rather they are not our focus.

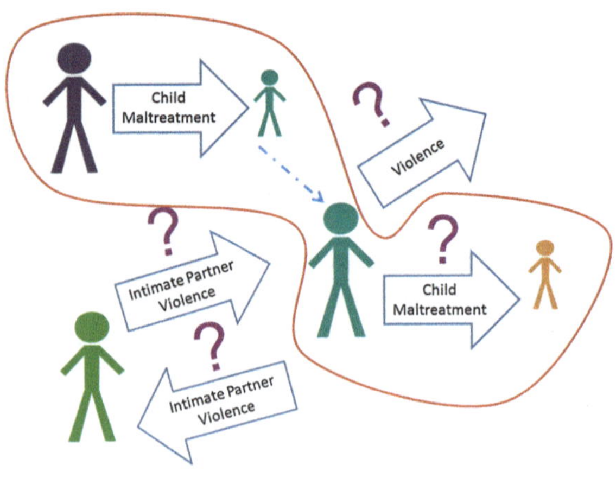

Fig. 1.1 Cycle of violence and intergenerational transmission of child maltreatment. This figure illustrates the cycle of violence and the relationship to the intergenerational transmission of child maltreatment which is highlighted within the circle

1.2 Scope of Child Maltreatment

Child maltreatment is an epidemic worldwide. According to the World Health Organization (2014), a quarter of adults report having been physically abused as children, and one in five women and one in 13 men report being sexually abused as a child. It is estimated that annually across the world there are 41,000 homicidal deaths of children under age 15, which underestimates the number of deaths due to maltreatment as death may wrongly be attributed to accidents (e.g., falls, drownings, burns) (World Health Organization 2014). There is growing recognition of the problem of child maltreatment. Currently, not all countries have child protection services and nongovernment organizations working to ensure the safety and well-being of children, and there is great variation among what is offered in individual countries (Sheeran 2008).

1.2.1 Child Maltreatment in the United States

In the United States, during fiscal year 2014, an estimated 3.6 million reports involving 6.6 million children were made to a child protection services agency (U.S. Department of Health and Human Services 2016). Of these reports, 2.2 million referrals (60.7 %) were screened-in with 3.2 million children receiving an investigation or alternative response. Including the 1580 fatalities, there were 702,000 victims. Almost two-thirds (63.7 %) of these children received post-response services as did almost one-third (32.0 %) of non-victims (U.S. Department of Health and Human Services 2016). It is important to note that a lack of substantiation does not necessarily mean maltreatment did not occur and that unsubstantiated cases are at risk for recidivism and future maltreatment (Kohl et al. 2009). Likewise, the reality of underreporting to child protective services cannot be overlooked. There may be groups that are underreported and it is widely accepted that the number of reports underestimate the prevalence of child abuse and neglect (Finkelhor 1994; MacMillan et al. 2003; U.S. Government Accountability Office 2011).

1.2.2 Impact of Child Maltreatment

While the numbers of children who are maltreated are staggering, they only tell part of the story. Children who experience abuse and neglect are at increased risk to face a wide range of poor outcomes across developmental, health, mental health, and social domains. Research has shown that maltreatment, especially extreme neglect, negatively impacts brain development at a young age (Teicher et al. 2003; Teicher et al. 2004; Twardosz and Lutzker 2010; Wilson et al. 2011). Children who are maltreated have lower cognitive development (Crozier and Barth 2005;

Jaffee and Maikovich-Fong 2011) as well as lower executive functioning than their peers (Beers and De Bellis 2002; De Bellis et al. 2009; DePrince et al. 2009; Prasad et al. 2005; Spann et al. 2012).

Abused and neglected children have higher rates of health problems including chronic health conditions (Flaherty et al. 2013; Nelson et al. 2011; Ringelsen et al. 2008). Likewise, maltreatment influences mental health. Adolescents who were abused as children are more likely to have mental health issues such as ADHD (Becker-Blease and Freyd 2008; Heneghan et al. 2013), conduct disorder (Fergusson et al. 2008; Kaplan et al. 1998), depression (Brown et al. 1999; Fergusson et al. 2008; Gilbert et al. 2009; Heneghan et al. 2013; Kaplan et al. 1998; Lansford et al. 2002), and posttraumatic stress disorder (Kearney et al. 2010; Kolko 2010).

Children who were maltreated are more likely than their peers to exhibit problems in their education and have less academic success (Crozier and Barth 2005; Eckenrode et al. 1993; Jaffee and Gallop 2007; Jonson-Reid et al. 2004). A history of child maltreatment is associated with problem behavior in adolescence (Gilbert et al. 2009; Lansford et al. 2002). Additionally, those who were maltreated as children, especially those who were sexually abused, are more likely to engage in earlier sexual behaviors (Noll et al. 2003; Wilson and Widom 2008) and high risk sexual behaviors (Lodico and DiClemente 1994; Noll et al. 2003; Senn et al. 2008) and are at risk for prostitution (Wilson and Widom 2010; Widom and Kuhns 1996).

The consequences and effects of maltreatment can last a lifetime. Children who were maltreated are more likely as adults to experience problems with health (Felitti et al. 1998; Herrenkohl et al. 2013; Wegman and Stetler 2009), mental health (Edwards et al. 2003; Fergusson et al. 2008; Gilbert et al. 2009; Herrenkohl et al. 2013; Widom 1998), substance use (Gilbert et al. 2009; Jonson-Reid et al. 2012; Herrenkohl et al. 2013; Kunitz et al. 1998), and intimate partner violence (Kunitz et al. 1998; Smith et al. 2011; Stith et al. 2000). Although those who were maltreated may be more likely than their peers to experience these problems, not all who have experienced maltreatment will go onto experience these negative outcomes. Researchers are working to identifying risk and protective factors for maltreatment. In Chaps. 4 and 5, we discuss risk and protective factors respectively as they pertain to ITCM.

Child maltreatment not only hurts children, but also it is costly to communities and all of society. It is estimated that child maltreatment lifetime costs per victim of nonfatal child maltreatment was $210,012 (in 2010 dollars) in the United States, taking into consideration medical expenses in childhood and adulthood, as well as the costs in the child welfare, criminal justice, and special education systems (Fang et al. 2012). The cost per death—$1,258,800—was estimated to be considerably higher considering losses in productivity. Taking into account the prevalence of child maltreatment, it should come as no surprise that the costs add up quickly. For new cases of both fatal and nonfatal child maltreatment in 2008 in the United States, the economic burden is approximately $124 billion (Fang et al. 2012).

1.3 Prevention and Intervention Strategies

Clearly, child maltreatment is costly after it occurs. Advocates for prevention argue that prevention could cost a small fraction of the amount of money being spent to address the consequences and aftermath of child maltreatment. Since child maltreatment was identified as a social problem, there has been prevention and intervention to address it. The Institute of Medicine and National Resource Council (2014) released a report "New Directions in Child Abuse and Neglect Research" that outlines priorities and sets the national agenda for research to reduce child maltreatment. It is widely accepted that for social and economic reasons, addressing child maltreatment requires urgent action.

It is imperative to develop strategies that stop maltreatment and promote well-being in children and families. The Centers for Disease Control and Prevention (CDC) has prioritized creating safe, stable, nurturing relationships and environments to prevent maltreatment and enhance well-being (CDC 2014). Chapter 7 focuses on prevention and intervention strategies.

1.3.1 Integrating Knowledge About Intergenerational Transmission of Child Maltreatment into Prevention and Intervention Strategies

To develop and assess child maltreatment prevention and intervention strategies, it is necessary to better understand ITCM. This means there is a need to critically examine the empirical evidence on ITCM and to have a stronger theoretical understanding of ITCM, as well as its risk and protective factors. This book attempts to pull together all of the threads and information to better understand what is known about ITCM and to organize the knowledge in a way that those conducting research and designing child maltreatment prevention and intervention strategies can use as a foundation.

1.4 Outline of the Book

This book synthesizes what is known about ITCM to guide those who are seeking information about child maltreatment and ITCM, as well as those who are developing interventions and conducting child maltreatment prevention research. The purpose of this book is to comprehensively review what is known about ITCM, critique the current literature, and offer direction for future research and interventions. The book is based on the premise that to effectively prevent child maltreatment, understanding the nature of ITCM is of utmost importance. The book is divided into seven chapters. The remaining chapters are described below.

1.4.1 Chapter 2: Theoretical Frameworks Conceptualizing Intergenerational Transmission of Child Maltreatment

Various theories have been used to understand child maltreatment and to guide the interventions and prevention of child maltreatment. This chapter presents different theoretical frameworks that are useful in understanding ITCM, including social learning theory, attachment theory, ecological models, and strengths and resilience frameworks. The conclusion highlights how risk and protective factors can guide the conceptualization and response to ITCM.

1.4.2 Chapter 3: Summary of Research on Intergenerational Transmission of Child Maltreatment

Over the past several decades, studies have examined ITCM using varying methods, variables, and samples. This chapter presents an organized and coherent description of these studies, both narratively and visually through a table to provide readers with an overview of research conducted on ITCM. The description of the studies includes type(s) of maltreatment examined; measurement of maltreatment; transmission rates of ITCM; and presence of risk, protective and contextual factors.

1.4.3 Chapter 4: Risk Factors Associated with Intergenerational Transmission of Child Maltreatment

This chapter is devoted to exploring the risk factors associated with ITCM. Relying on empirical studies about child maltreatment and ITCM, this chapter highlights several risk factors of ITCM, including individual characteristics related to the parents (e.g., substance abuse, mental health, and early parenting) and child (e.g., disability), family circumstances (e.g., family structure, parenting skills, and intimate partner violence), and contextual factors (e.g., poverty, neighborhoods). The chapter discusses the complexity of risk and co-occurring factors and the challenges associated with the relationship between the factors and ITCM.

1.4.4 Chapter 5: Interrupting Intergenerational Transmission of Child Maltreatment: Protective Factors Associated with Breaking the Cycle of Maltreatment

This chapter discusses resilience and protective factors and their importance when examining ITCM. Several factors have been identified in the child maltreatment literature as having the potential to buffer the negative outcomes associated with child maltreatment and ITCM. These factors include education, social support, positive relationships, resources, and resilience. This chapter includes a discussion of protective factors shown to reduce ITCM as well as other potential factors that have not yet been fully explored.

1.4.5 Chapter 6: Future Research on Intergenerational Transmission of Child Maltreatment: Methods, Constructs, and Contexts

This chapter presents the ways, contexts, and populations with which ITCM has been studied. It describes the limitations of current studies on ITCM and the need for improved methods. It argues that there is still much to be discovered in terms of how ITCM is related to various constructs and contexts, such as poverty, intimate partner violence, trauma, and mental health. There are few, if any, studies specifically examining ITCM within these contexts or within specific populations such as child welfare involved children and families, youth who are aging out of the child welfare system, and across cultures. This chapter offers specific recommendations for future research within these contexts and others related to ITCM. This chapter begins with an introduction to previously proposed methodological standards for evaluating ITCM and leads to a description of how this information can be used to guide future studies.

1.4.6 Chapter 7: Prevention and Intervention Strategies to Address Intergenerational Transmission of Child Maltreatment

In order to better understand child maltreatment and to be able to develop useful and effective interventions to prevent child maltreatment, greater understanding of intergenerational transmission of child maltreatment (ITCM) is necessary along with the contexts in which it occurs. This chapter examines specific populations that have been identified who may be at a greater risk of ITCM as well as interventions proposed to interrupt ITCM. Populations such as child welfare involved families may be disproportionally affected by ITCM. Families and individuals experiencing trauma may also be at greater risk. Various interventions have been developed to address the risks associated with child maltreatment and can be adapted to special populations and families affected by or at greater risk of intergenerational maltreatment. The chapter concludes with recommendations for continued rigorous evaluation of intervention and prevention strategies.

References

Becker-Blease, K. A., & Freyd, J. J. (2008). A preliminary study of ADHD symptoms and correlates: Do abused children differ from nonabused children? *Journal of Aggression, Maltreatment and Trauma, 17*, 133–140.

Beers, S. R., & De Bellis, M. D. (2002). Neuropsychological function in children with maltreatment-related posttraumatic stress disorder. *American Journal of Psychiatry, 159*, 483–486.

Berlin, L. J., Appleyard, K., & Dodge, K. A. (2011). Intergenerational continuity in child maltreatment: Mediating mechanisms and implications for prevention. *Child Development, 82*(1), 162–176.

Brown, J., Cohen, P., Johnson, J. G., & Smailes, E. M. (1999). Childhood abuse and neglect: Specificity of effects on adolescent and young adult depression and suicidality. *Journal of the American Academy of Child and Adolescent Psychiatry, 38*, 1490–1496.

Centers for Disease Control and Prevention. (2014). Essentials for childhood: Steps to create safe, stable, nurturing relationships and environments. Retrieved from http://www.cdc.gov/violenceprevention/pdf/essentials_for_childhood_framework.pdf

Child Abuse Prevention and Treatment Act as amended by P.L. 111–320. The CAPTA Reauthorization Act of 2010, 42 U.S.C. § 5106(g).

Crozier, J. C., & Barth, R. P. (2005). Cognitive and academic functioning in maltreated children. *Children & Schools, 27*(4), 197–206.

De Bellis, M. D., Hooper, S. R., Spratt, E. G., & Woolley, D. P. (2009). Neuropsychological findings in childhood neglect and their relationships to pediatric PTSD. *Journal of the International Neuropsychological Society, 15*, 868–878.

DePrince, A. P., Weinzierl, K. M., & Combs, M. D. (2009). Executive function performance and trauma exposure in a community sample of children. *Child Abuse and Neglect, 33*, 353–361.

Dixon, L., Browne, K., & Hamilton-Giachritsis, C. (2009). Patterns of risk and protective factors in the intergenerational cycle of maltreatment. *Journal of Family Violence, 24*(2), 111–122.

Eckenrode, J., Laird, M., & Doris, J. (1993). School performance and disciplinary problems among abused and neglected children. *Developmental Psychology, 29*, 53–62.

Edwards, V. J., Holden, G. W., Felitti, V. J., & Anda, R. F. (2003). Relationship between multiple forms of childhood maltreatment and adult mental health in community respondents: Results from the adverse childhood experiences study. *American Journal of Psychiatry, 160*(8), 1453–1460.

Egeland, B., Jacobvitz, D., & Sroufe, L. A. (1988). Breaking the cycle of abuse. *Child Development, 59*(4), 1080–1088.

Ertem, I. O., Leventhal, J. M., & Dobbs, S. (2000). Intergenerational continuity of child physical abuse: How good is the evidence? *The Lancet, 356*(9232), 814–819.

Fang, X., Brown, D. S., Florence, C. S., & Mercy, J. A. (2012). The economic burden of child maltreatment in the United States and implications for prevention. *Child Abuse and Neglect, 36*(2), 156–165.

Felitti, V. J., Anda, R. F., Nordenberg, D., Williamson, D. F., Spitz, A. M., Edwards, V., et al. (1998). Relationship of childhood abuse and household dysfunction to many of the leading causes of death in adults: The Adverse Childhood Experiences (ACE) Study. *American Journal of Preventive Medicine, 14*, 245–258.

Fergusson, D. M., Boden, J. M., & Horwood, L. J. (2008). Exposure to childhood sexual and physical abuse and adjustment in early adulthood. *Child Abuse and Neglect, 32*, 607–619.

Finkelhor, D. (1994). Current information on the scope and nature of child sexual abuse. *The Future of Children, 4*, 31–53.

Flaherty, E. G., Thompson, R., Dubowitz, H., Harvey, E., English, D. J., Proctor, L. J., et al. (2013). Adverse childhood experiences and child health in early adolescence. *Pediatrics, 167*, 622–629.

Garbarino, J., & Gilliam, G. (1980). *Understanding abusive families*. Lexington, MA: Lexington Books.

Gilbert, R., Widom, C. S., Browne, K., Fergusson, D., Webb, E., & Janson, S. (2009). Burden and consequences of child maltreatment in high-income countries. *The Lancet, 37*, 68–81.

Heneghan, A., Stein, R. E. K., Hurlburt, M. S., Zhang, J., Rolls-Reutz, J., Fisher, E., et al. (2013). Mental health problems in teens investigated by U.S. child welfare agencies. *Journal of Adolescent Health, 52*, 634–640.

Herrenkohl, T. I., Hong, S., Klika, J. B., Herrenkohl, R. C., & Russo, M. J. (2013). Developmental impacts of child abuse and neglect related to adult mental health, substance use, and physical health. *Journal of Family Violence, 28*(2), 191–199.

Heyman, R. E., & Slep, A. M. S. (2002). Do child abuse and interparental violence lead to adulthood family violence?. *Journal of Marriage and Family, 64*(4), 864–870.

Hubbard, D. J., & Pratt, T. C. (2002). A meta-analysis of the predictors of delinquency among girls. *Journal of Offender Rehabilitation, 34*, 1–13.

Institute of Medicine & National Research Council. (2014). *New directions in child abuse and neglect research*. Washington, DC: The National Academies Press.

Jaffee, S. R., & Gallop, R. (2007). Social, emotional, and academic competence among children who have had contact with child protective services: Prevalence and stability estimates. *Journal of the American Academy of Child and Adolescent Psychiatry, 46*, 757–765.

Jaffee, S. R., & Maikovich-Fong, A. K. (2011). Effects of chronic maltreatment and maltreatment timing on children's behavior and cognitive abilities. *Journal of Child Psychology and Psychiatry and Allied Disciplines, 52*, 184–194.

Jonson-Reid, M., Drake, B., Kim, J. S., Porterfield, S., & Han, L. (2004). A prospective analysis of the relationship between reported child maltreatment and special education eligibility among poor children. *Child Maltreatment, 9*, 382–394.

Jonson-Reid, M., Kohl, P. L., & Drake, B. (2012). Child and adult outcomes of chronic child maltreatment. *Pediatrics, 129*, 839–845.

Kaplan, S. J., Pelcovitz, D., Salzinger, S., Weiner, M., Mandel, F. S., Lesser, M. L., et al. (1998). Adolescent physical abuse: Risk for adolescent psychiatric disorders. *American Journal of Psychiatry, 155*, 954–959.

Kaufman, J., & Zigler, E. (1987). Do abused children become abusive parents? *American Journal of Orthopsychiatry, 57*(2), 186.

Kearney, C. A., Wechsler, A., Kaur, H., & Lemos-Miller, A. (2010). Posttraumatic stress disorder in maltreated youth: A review of contemporary research and thought. *Clinical Child and Family Psychology Review, 13*, 46–76.

Kim, J. (2009). Type-specific intergenerational transmission of neglectful and physically abusive parenting behaviors among young parents. *Children and Youth Services Review, 31*(7), 761–767.

Kohl, P. L., Jonson-Reid, M., & Drake, B. (2009). Time to leave substantiation behind findings from a national probability study. *Child Maltreatment, 14*, 17–26.

Kolko, D. J. (2010). Posttraumatic stress symptoms in children and adolescents referred for child welfare investigation a national sample of in-home and out-of-home care. *Child Maltreatment, 15*, 48–63.

Kunitz, S. J., Levy, J. E., McCloskey, J., & Gabriel, K. R. (1998). Alcohol dependence and domestic violence as sequelae of abuse and conduct disorder in childhood. *Child Abuse and Neglect, 22*(11), 1079–1091.

Lansford, J. E., Dodge, K. A., Pettit, G. S., Bates, J. E., Crozier, J., & Kaplow, J. (2002). A 12-year prospective study of the long-term effects of early child physical maltreatment on psychological, behavioral, and academic problems in adolescence. *Archives of Pediatrics and Adolescent Medicine, 156*, 824–830.

Lansford, J. E., Miller-Johnson, S., Berlin, L. J., Dodge, K. A., Bates, J. E., & Pettit, G. S. (2007). Early physical abuse and later violent delinquency: A prospective longitudinal study. *Child Maltreatment, 12*, 233–245.

Lodico, M. A., & DiClemente, R. J. (1994). The association between childhood sexual abuse and prevalence of HIV-related risk behaviors. *Clinical Pediatrics, 33*, 498–502.

MacMillan, H. L., Jamieson, E., & Walsh, C. A. (2003). Reported contact with child protection services among those reporting child physical and sexual abuse: Results from a community survey. *Child Abuse and Neglect, 27*, 1397–1408.

Marshall, J. M., Huang, H., & Ryan, J. P. (2011). Intergenerational families in child welfare: Assessing needs and estimating permanency. *Children and Youth Services Review, 33*(6), 1024–1030.

Maxfield, M. G., & Widom, C. S. (1996). The cycle of violence: Revisited 6 years later. *Archives of Pediatrics and Adolescent Medicine, 150*, 390–395.

McKinney, C. M., Caetano, R., Ramisetty-Mikler, S., & Nelson, S. (2009). Childhood family violence and perpetration and victimization of intimate partner violence: Findings from a national population-based study of couples. *Annals of Epidemiology, 19*(1), 25–32.

Nelson, T. D., Smith, T. R., Thompson, R. W., Epstein, M. H., Griffith, A. K., Hurley, K. D., et al. (2011). Prevalence of physical health problems among youth entering residential treatment. *Pediatrics, 128*, e1226–e1232.

Noll, J. G., Trickett, P. K., & Putnam, F. W. (2003). A prospective investigation of the impact of childhood sexual abuse on the development of sexuality. *Journal of Consulting and Clinical Psychology, 71*, 575–586.

Pears, K. C., & Capaldi, D. M. (2001). Intergenerational transmission of abuse: A two-generational prospective study of an at-risk sample. *Child Abuse and Neglect, 25*(11), 1439–1461.

Prasad, M. R., Kramer, L. A., & Ewing-Cobbs, L. (2005). Cognitive and neuroimaging findings in physically abused preschoolers. *Archive of Disease in Childhood, 90*, 82–85.

Renner, L. M., & Slack, K. S. (2006). Intimate partner violence and child maltreatment: Understanding intra-and intergenerational connections. *Child Abuse and Neglect, 30*(6), 599–617.

Ringelsen, H., Casanueva, C., Urato, M., & Cross, T. (2008). Special health care needs among children in the child welfare system. *Pediatrics, 122*, e232–e241.

Rivera, B., & Widom, C. S. (1990). Childhood victimization and violent offending. *Violence and Victims, 5*(1), 19–35.

Schwartz, I. M., Rendon, J. A., & Hsieh, C. M. (1994). Is child maltreatment a leading cause of delinquency? *Child Welfare, 73*, 639.

Senn, T., Carey, M. P., & Vanable, P. A. (2008). Childhood and adolescent sexual abuse and subsequent sexual risk behavior: Evidence from controlled studies, methodological critique, and suggestions for research. *Clinical Psychology Review, 28*, 711–735.

Sheeran, A. (2008). *UNICEF child protection meta-evaluation*. New York: Child Protection Section, Programme Division, United Nations Children's Fund.

Sidebotham, P., Heron, J., & ALSPAC Study Team. (2006). Child maltreatment in the "children of the nineties": A cohort study of risk factors. *Child Abuse & Neglect, 30*(5), 497–522.

Smith, C. A., Ireland, T. O., Park, A., Elwyn, L., & Thornberry, T. P. (2011). Intergenerational continuities and discontinuities in intimate partner violence: A two-generation prospective study. *Journal of Interpersonal Violence, 26*, 3720–3752.

Smith, C. A., Ireland, T. O., & Thornberry, T. P. (2005). Adolescent maltreatment and its impact on young adult antisocial behavior. *Child Abuse and Neglect, 29*, 1099–1119.

Smith, C., & Thornberry, T. P. (1995). The relationship between childhood maltreatment and adolescent involvement in delinquency. *Criminology, 33*, 451–481.

Spann, M. N., Mayes, L. C., Kalmar, J. H., Guiney, J., Womer, F. Y., Pittman, B., et al. (2012). Childhood abuse and neglect and cognitive flexibility in adolescents. *Child Neuropsychology, 18*, 182–189.

Stith, S. M., Rosen, K. H., Middleton, K. A., Busch, A. L., Lundeberg, K., & Carlton, R. P. (2000). The intergenerational transmission of spouse abuse: A meta-analysis. *Journal of Marriage and Family, 62*(3), 640–654.

Stouthamer-Loeber, M., Loeber, R., Homish, D. L., & Wei, E. (2001). Maltreatment of boys and the development of disruptive and delinquent behavior. *Development and Psychopathology, 13*, 941–955.

Teicher, M. H., Andersen, S. L., Polcari, A., Anderson, C. M., Navalta, C. P., & Kim, D. M. (2003). The neurobiological consequences of early stress and childhood maltreatment. *Neuroscience and Biobehavioral Reviews, 27*(1), 33–44.

Teicher, M. H., Dumont, N. L., Ito, Y., Vaituzis, C., Giedd, J. N., & Andersen, S. L. (2004). Childhood neglect is associated with reduced corpus callosum area. *Biological Psychiatry, 56*(2), 80–85.

Thornberry, T. P., Knight, K. E., & Lovegrove, P. J. (2012). Does maltreatment beget maltreatment? A systematic review of the intergenerational literature. *Trauma, Violence, & Abuse, 13*(3), 135–152.

Twardosz, S., & Lutzker, J. R. (2010). Child maltreatment and the developing brain: A review of neuroscience perspectives. *Aggression and Violent Behavior, 15*, 59–68.

U.S. Department of Health and Human Services, Administration for Children and Families, Administration on Children, Youth and Families, Children's Bureau. (2016). Child maltreatment 2014. Available from http://www.acf.hhs.gov/programs/cb/resource/child-maltreatment-2014

U.S. Government Accountability Office. (2011). *Child maltreatment: Strengthening national data on child fatalities could aid in prevention*. Washington, DC: Government Accountability Office.

Valentino, K., Nutall, A. K., Comas, M., Borkowski, J. G., & Akai, C. E. (2012). Intergenerational continuity of child abuse among adolescent mothers: Authoritarian parenting, community violence, and race. *Child Maltreatment, 17*(2), 172–181.

Wegman, H. L., & Stetler, C. (2009). A meta-analytic review of the effects of childhood abuse on medical outcomes in adulthood. *Psychosomatic Medicine, 71*(8), 805–812.

White, H. R., & Widom, C. S. (2003). Intimate partner violence among abused and neglected children in young adulthood: The mediating effects of early aggression, antisocial personality, hostility and alcohol problems. *Aggressive Behavior, 29*(4), 332–345.

Widom, C. S. (1989a). Child abuse, neglect, and adult behavior: Research design and findings on criminality, violence, and child abuse. *American Journal of Orthopsychiatry, 59*(3), 355–367.

Widom, C. S. (1989b). Child abuse, neglect, and violent criminal behavior. *Criminology, 27*(2), 251–271.

Widom, C. S. (1989c). Does violence beget violence? A critical examination of the literature. *Psychological Bulletin, 106*(1), 3–28.

Widom, C. S. (1998). Child victims: Searching for opportunities to break the cycle of violence. *Applied and Preventive Psychology, 7*(4), 225–234.

Widom, C. S., Czaja, S., & Dutton, M. A. (2014). Child abuse and neglect and intimate partner violence victimization and perpetration: A prospective investigation. *Child Abuse and Neglect, 38*(4), 650–663.

Widom, C. S., & Kuhns, J. B. (1996). Childhood victimization and subsequent risk for promiscuity, prostitution, and teenage pregnancy: A prospective study. *American Journal of Public Health, 86*, 1607–1612.

Widom, C. S., & Wilson, H. W. (2015). Intergenerational transmission of violence. In J. Lindert & I. Levav (Eds.), *Violence and mental health* (pp. 27–45). Netherlands: Springer.

Wilson, K. R., Hansen, D. J., & Li, M. (2011). The traumatic stress response in child maltreatment and resultant neuropsychological effects. *Aggression and Violent Behavior, 16*(2), 87–97.

Wilson, H. W., & Widom, C. S. (2008). An examination of risky sexual behavior and HIV in victims of child abuse and neglect: A 30-year follow-up. *Health Psychology, 27*(2), 149.

Wilson, H. W., & Widom, C. S. (2010). The role of youth problem behaviors in the path from child abuse and neglect to prostitution: A prospective examination. *Journal of Research on Adolescence, 20*(1), 210–236.

World Health Organization. (2014). *Child maltreatment.* Retrieved from http://www.who.int/mediacentre/factsheets/fs150/en

Chapter 2
Theoretical Frameworks Conceptualizing Intergenerational Transmission of Child Maltreatment

2.1 Conceptualizing Intergenerational Transmission of Child Maltreatment

Since the 1960s, several major theories and frameworks have been used to explain child maltreatment, such as psychodynamic/psychopathology framework, Social Learning Theory, Attachment Theory, ecological models, strengths and resilience frameworks, and Social Information Processing Theory. These theories and frameworks have implications for the Intergenerational Transmission of Child Maltreatment (ITCM), and scholars have used them individually and in combination to examine ITCM. This chapter presents different theoretical frameworks that are useful in understanding ITCM along with some of the limitations.

2.2 Psychodynamic Models

Early research identified parental psychopathology as the cause of child maltreatment that needed to be treated psychiatrically (Ammerman 1990). There was little empirical support for this theoretical view and it was flawed with methodological issues. The model was criticized when studies showed that only a small percentage of maltreating parents actually experienced any psychopathological disorder (Kempe et al. 1985). However, some specific forms of parental psychopathology are risk factors for child maltreatment (Institute of Medicine and National Resource Council 2014). Maternal depression and anxiety have been associated with physical abuse and neglect (Brown et al. 1998). Antisocial personality disorders are also a risk factor (Belsky and Vondra 1989).

While ITCM research has not been driven by the belief that parental psychopathology causes child maltreatment, mental health variables have been

L. Schelbe and J.M. Geiger, *Intergenerational Transmission of Child Maltreatment*, SpringerBriefs in Social Work,
DOI 10.1007/978-3-319-43824-5_2

incorporated into studies. It has been argued that the consequences of child maltreatment such as mental health issues function as risk factors for the cycle of maltreatment continuing (Frias-Armenta 2002). Several studies found that depressive symptoms linked a history of child maltreatment and perpetrating child maltreatment (Banyard et al. 2003; Dixon et al. 2005a, b; Pears and Capaldi 2001; Thompson 2006). Dixon and colleagues (2005a) found parental mental illness/depression partially mediated ITCM. Jaffee and colleagues (2013) found the mothers in their study sample with a history of child maltreatment were more likely to have mental health problems, and those with a history of maltreatment who maltreated their children experienced more depression and antisocial behavior.

2.3 Social Learning Theory

Social Learning Theory is primarily concerned with an individual's learning through cognitive processes, modeling, and social observation (Bandura 1977). The basic principle is that humans can learn through observing models. Social Learning Theory provides a framework for understanding child maltreatment, especially in terms of its transmission across generations. For example, if a child experiences violence or maltreatment from a parent, the child learns that this is an acceptable interaction and may in turn imitate or exhibit similar behavior within similar and other situations. Behavior can also be reinforced through observation of rewards and punishments following the behavior. Social Learning Theory has been used to understand patterns of child maltreatment among individuals who have experienced abuse and/or neglect themselves as children. It is believed that children learn adaptive and maladaptive parenting practices from their own experiences of being parented. It could also be argued that the lack of a positive parenting model could cause a person to be unaware of necessary parenting skills to care for a child, potentially causing harm or neglect. The relationship between childhood history of abuse and the perpetration of abuse/neglect has been established; however, there is no causal link, and a history of abuse is not a necessary factor, nor is it the only factor. Social Learning Theory also fails to acknowledge many of the environmental factors that may shape parenting attitudes and contribute to child maltreatment and ITCM.

Studies examining ITCM both explicitly and implicitly incorporate Social Learning Theory. The transmission process is often implicitly based in Social Learning Theory. Studies may not necessarily cite Social Learning Theory, but they use terms that are consistent with Social Learning Theory such as "learned behavior" and "behavior modeling." However, some scholars explicitly ground their studies within Social Learning Theory (e.g., Marshall et al. 2011; Renner and Slack 2006; Widom and Wilson 2015).

2.4 Social Information Processing Theory

Social Information Processing Theory is concerned with all of the mental operations that are deployed to generate a behavioral response during social interaction. The theory seeks to understand how behavior results from peoples' understanding and interacting with their surroundings. The mental operations that are considered include selective attention to social cues, attribution of intent, generation of goals, accessing of behavioral scripts from memory, decision-making, and behavioral enactment. There are five stages that progresses where information is obtained and processed that ultimately leads to action. The stages are encoding, creating mental representations, response accessing, evaluation, and enactment.

Social Information Processing Theory has implications for understanding child maltreatment (Milner 1993, 2003). Specifically, researchers have examined social information processing as it relates to aggressive behavior of children who have been maltreated (Burks et al. 1999; Dodge et al. 1990) as well as their social adaptation (Price and Landsverk 1998). Studies have also used social information processing as the foundation of studies examining how parents perceive children's behaviors and attributes (Dadds et al. 2003; Montes et al. 2001). For example, Montes et al. (2001) compared mothers at low risk and high risk for child maltreatment and found evidence for social information processing of child physical abuse. They concluded that mothers in the two different groups processed information related to children differently and used more power-assertive discipline.

As Social Information Processing Theory has been used to examine both the outcomes of children who have been maltreated and parents who are at risk for maltreating their children, the theory can be seen as relevant to ITCM. When examining ITCM, Berlin and colleagues (2011) used Social Information Processing Theory to understand how we behave based on how we selectively attend to and respond to social cues. Berlin and colleagues (2011) conducted research to better understand aggression, child maltreatment, and ITCM through how individuals cognitively process social cues and act on their understanding of others and their behavior. Scholars believe that it is possible that children who experience physical maltreatment may be more likely to develop "biased patterns of processing social information" (Berlin et al. 2011, p. 164). Kim (2012) compares Social Information Processing Theory with Nisbett's Cultural Cognitive Theory and Turiel's Social-Cognitive Domain Theory to understand the role of culture in the intergenerational transmission of violence.

2.5 Attachment Theory

Attachment between a child and caregiver begins at birth when a child is completely dependent on the caregiver for survival and relies on the caregiver to provide consistent and responsive care. Through this process, an attachment is formed between the child and the caregiver that is reciprocal in nature, where a behavior from one evokes a response from the other. For example, a hungry child cries and the caregiver responds either by meeting the child's needs or not. According to Attachment Theory, the attachment relationship which continues through the first years of a child's life serves as the template for future relationships and interactions in the social world (Bowlby 1982). Attachment security is the basis for a child's psychological growth and the development of mental representations that are subsequently applied to the child's current and future environment (Bowlby 1982). The attachment between caregiver and child becomes the foundation for the child to develop a sense of trust and security, a sense of self, and an ability to explore his/her environment (Ainsworth 1989; Bowlby 1982). When a secure attachment is not established between the caregiver and child, a child may develop an internal working model that reflects an inconsistency and unresponsiveness in others that translates into unrealistic expectations of others. The child may also experience adverse developmental consequences related to physical, behavioral, cognitive, and social functioning, such as aggressive behavior.

Attachment Theory helps us understand how individuals with a history of child maltreatment can experience various challenges related to interpersonal relationships, parenting, and psychosocial functioning in adulthood. Maltreated children may experience instability in the home, distant and inconsistent parenting, and inconsistent supervision and discipline. Children who have been abused and neglected tend to show insecure–avoidant attachment patterns and may experience difficulty in future intimate relationships (Baer and Martinez 2006; Crittenden 1992; Hildyard and Wolfe 2002). It might then be postulated that maltreated children who have experienced a dysfunctional attachment may then display similar attachment patterns with their children and others. Research has shown that parents who experienced childhood maltreatment may have inconsistent parenting patterns and the children of parents who have experienced maltreatment and poor attachment with their caregivers exhibit the same parenting behaviors, possibly placing their children at risk of maltreatment (Robboy and Anderson 2011).

Despite the relevance of Attachment Theory in understanding the experiences of maltreated children, methods in measuring and testing this theory have significant limitations. Youth and adults have a difficult time recalling their own attachment experiences as infants and young children, and most interactions between caregiver and child are experienced privately and are difficult to observe in a natural environment. Another limitation in the application of Attachment Theory to child maltreatment is that cultural differences are often not considered in experimental studies and/or when determining what constitutes 'normal' parent–child interactions. In addition, most of the research in attachment in the 1970s and 80s was conducted with mothers as caregivers with young toddlers and did not include fathers, grandparents, siblings, or other caring adults in the child's life.

Considering the importance of attachment and relationships as they relate to ITCM, measuring and documenting these patterns has been lacking in the ITCM research literature. An exception is Egeland and colleagues (1988) who used Attachment Theory in their examination of mothers who were maltreated as children and found that those who received emotional support from a nonabusive adult during childhood were more likely than the mothers who did not receive emotional support during childhood to break the cycle of abuse. Zuravin and colleagues (1996) also examined attachment and found that parents who experience maltreatment as children and had poor quality attachments with their caregivers were more likely than those with quality attachments to maltreat their children. Lounds and colleagues (2006) provided one of the more comprehensive uses of Attachment Theory in their ITCM study through using video interactions between mother and child to assess parent–child attachment. More recently, Thornberry and colleagues (2013) examined parent–child attachment as a protective factor in ITCM, although there was no evidence that attachment served as a protective factor. Thus, there is some support for attachment playing a role in ITCM. While scholars have identified Attachment Theory as a construct that can help understand ITCM, empirical studies have not adequately applied the theory.

2.6 Ecological Models

The ecological perspective posits that humans are active in the developmental process and are constantly affecting and being affected by their environment (Bronfenbrenner 1979; Bronfenbrenner and Morris 2006). Brofenbrenner's (1979) ecological model typically involves four types of systems that interact and contain distinct but related roles, norms and rules, each nested within the next, that influence development and behavior: the microsystem, the mesosystem, the exosystem, and the macrosystem. The nature of the parent–child relationship is dependent on the interaction between factors in the child's and the parents' maturing biology, the immediate family and community environment, as well as the social landscape.

In order to capture the multidimensional concepts of parenting, child maltreatment, and ITCM, Bronfenbrenner's (1979) ecological model is a helpful and commonly used framework to understand ITCM (e.g., Leve et al. 2015; Sidebotham 2001; Valentino et al. 2012). Within this context, the microsystem is the individual (as parent or child) and the individuals' resources and characteristics that impact parenting. For example, the parent's, in addition to the child's, disposition and temperament will influence parental functioning. The mesosystem refers to the individual's active interaction within microsystems or the connections between contexts. The exosystem includes the link between a social setting in which the individual does not have an active role, nor is it within the individual's immediate surroundings (Bronfenbrenner 1979). For example, the relationship between family experiences and school or church experiences is part of the mesosystem, while the exosystem includes support networks and influences as well as the social context to which the parent has been exposed. The mesosystem and exosystem consist of the immediate family and household, as well as the systems in which the individual and/or family are embedded. Finally, the macrosystem consists of larger cultural and societal influences with the individual being active in interactions with the social network and establishing the norms within this group. The macro level influences on child maltreatment and parental attitudes include cultural beliefs, the media, racism, as well as educational and economic opportunities. Family circumstances such as socioeconomic status, lack of social support, and neighborhood factors associated with child maltreatment and ITCM may have a direct or indirect effect on parenting ability, and these circumstances can act as risks or protective factors.

Belsky's (1984) Process Model of Parenting uses an ecological perspective in describing the individual and environmental factors that contribute to parenting practices. The model proposes that parenting practices are multiply determined by and nested within (a) the parent, (b) the child, and (c) the larger socio-cultural context of the parent and child. In Belsky's (1984) model, parent characteristics include the parent's developmental history and personality. A mature and healthy personality and positive experiences of being parented as a child might elicit sensitive parenting characteristics. Child characteristics, such as behavior and temperament, can influence the quality and quantity of parental responses. Parents may also experience a certain degree of stress from sources in the social environment, such as work and/or marriage. Belsky (1984) believed that parental characteristics and positive social supports have more influence on parenting than do child characteristics. He noted, for example, that difficult infant temperament does not compromise the quality of parenting if the parent has adequate supports and resources.

The use of an ecological framework has proved to be helpful in developing a greater understanding of various social phenomena with its ability to incorporate multiple levels of influences and interactions. Critics, however, suggest that Bronfenbrenner's ecological model is extremely broad and very difficult to test, and that it is perhaps instead a meta-theory that can essentially be applied to any concept or issue. Despite this, ecological models are used to provide a more comprehensive and descriptive approach and guide to child maltreatment assessment and interventions.

It is difficult to examine child maltreatment and ITCM within the context of either the individual or the environment. Child maltreatment and ITCM cannot be fully explained by one or the other, and a more complete understanding emerges only when the interactions of multiple levels of individual and familial characteristics, and the environment are examined simultaneously. Some examples presented in the research on child maltreatment and the formation of parenting attitudes and practices with an ecological framework include earlier works of Belsky (1993, 1984) and Baumrind (1994). Baumrind (1994) used an ecological perspective to unearth the impact of the social context in child maltreatment, specifically highlighting the economic and cultural factors that affect the occurrence of child maltreatment. Sidebotham (2001) outlined explicitly how an ecological approach can be used to examine child maltreatment and ITCM. More recently, Li and colleagues (2011), Currie and Widom (2010), and Dubowitz and colleagues (2011) used an ecological framework in examining long term consequences of child abuse and neglect, protective factors among families at risk of child maltreatment, and identifying children who are at high risk of child maltreatment and ITCM. Kotchick and

Forehand (2002) also contend that the use of an ecological perspective allows us to conceptualize "parenting as a process…that will facilitate a more sensitive approach to interventions and public policies" (p. 256). An ecological perspective allows for a multidimensional approach to understanding parenting, child maltreatment, and ITCM and is most appropriate in guiding study's research questions, methodology, and analysis.

2.7 Strengths and Resilience Frameworks

Human service professionals, social workers, and other helping professionals are often charged with assisting children and families in challenging situations. With the violence, oppression, poverty, and disease that many of the children and families face, it can be difficult to focus on strengths, the positive side of life, and how they are able to manage and overcome many of the challenges they face. However, it has been shown to be clinically beneficial for clients and professionals to focus more on strengths—individual, family, and community related positive attributes, skills, and accomplishments—instead of only managing the difficulties. As discussed in Chaps. 4 and 5, it is helpful for researchers and practitioners to study and acknowledge the risk factors associated with one's condition and experiences. However, it is equally important to also acknowledge, focus on, and cultivate the protective factors and resiliency one possesses.

Similarly, in examining and understanding ITCM, in addition to understanding the risks associated with ITCM, we must continue to focus on the strengths associated with how and when ITCM does not occur. Oftentimes, individuals possess a number of individual, familial, and community strengths and resources that they draw on to help with breaking the cycle of ITCM. Several of the studies presented and discussed in this text do not explicitly identify a theoretical framework guiding their research; however, many identify risk and protective factors and examine their influence on ITCM (e.g., Brown et al. 1998; Berlin et al. 2011). For more of a discussion on risk and resilience factors associated with ITCM, see Chaps. 4 and 5.

2.8 Combination of Theoretical Frameworks

In examining ITCM, several scholars use a combination of theoretical frameworks to better understand the risk and protective factors as well as the pathways of ITCM. For example, Marshall and colleagues (2011) applied Attachment Theory, Social Learning Theory, and socioecological models to better understand the parent, family, and child factors that play a role in ITCM. Widom and Wilson (2015) combined Social Learning Theory, Attachment Theory, Social Information Processing, neurophysiological models, and behavioral genetics to guide their research. Ben-David and colleagues (2015) propose several theories to inform their study, such as trauma and stress theories, psychopathology, and social learning theory. All of these scholars who grounded their studies in theoretical frameworks select variables and outcomes suggested not only by previous research, but also from theory.

2.9 Conclusion

Researchers and practitioners alike use a variety of theoretical frameworks in understanding human behavior, and in this case, the context and dynamics of ITCM. Using a theoretical framework helps guide our research and practice as well as helps to organize new and emerging ideas and knowledge. Several things can drive our choice of framework, such as experience, training, orientation, and research questions. It is helpful to be aware of how ITCM is being conceptualized, researched, and understood by others. Based on the framework used, intervention efforts can be structured differently. This chapter is not all encompassing, but presents a brief overview of many of the theoretical frameworks that have been used to better understanding ITCM.

References

Ainsworth, M. S. (1989). Attachments beyond infancy. *American Psychologist, 44*(4), 709.

Ammerman, R. T. (1990). Etiological models of child maltreatment a behavioral perspective. *Behavior Modification, 14*(3), 230–254.

Bandura, A. (1977). *Social learning theory*. Englewood Cliffs: Prentice-Hall.

Baer, J. C., & Martinez, C. D. (2006). Child maltreatment and insecure attachment: A meta-analysis. *Journal of Reproductive and Infant Psychology, 24*(3), 187–197.

Banyard, V. L., Williams, L. M., & Siegel, J. A. (2003). The impact of complex trauma and depression on parenting: An exploration of mediating risk and protective factors. *Child Maltreatment, 8*(4), 334–349.

Baumrind, D. (1994). The social context of child maltreatment. *Family Relations* 360–368.

Belsky, J. (1984). The determinants of parenting: A process model. *Child Development* 83–96.

Belsky, J. (1993). Etiology of child maltreatment: A developmental Ecological analysis. *Psychological Bulletin, 114*(3), 413.

Belsky, J., & Vondra, J. (1989). Lessons from child abuse: The determinants of parenting. In Cicchetti & V. Carlson (Eds.), *Child maltreatment: Theory and research on the causes and consequences of child abuse and neglect*. Cambridge, UK: Cambridge University Press.

Ben-David, V., Jonson-Reid, M., Drake, B., & Kohl, P. (2015). The association between childhood maltreatment experiences and the onset of maltreatment perpetration in young adulthood controlling for proximal and distal factors. *Child Abuse and Neglect, 46*, 132–141.

Berlin, L. J., Appleyard, K., & Dodge, K. A. (2011). Intergenerational continuity in child maltreatment: Mediating mechanisms and implications for prevention. *Child Development, 82*(1), 162–176.

Bowlby, J. (1982). Attachment and loss: retrospect and prospect. *American Journal of Orthopsychiatry, 52*(4), 664.

Bronfenbrenner, U. (1979). Contexts of child rearing: Problems and prospects. *American Psychologist, 34*(10), 844.
Bronfenbrenner, U., & Morris, P. A. (2006). The bioecological model of human development. *Handbook of child psychology*.
Brown, J., Cohen, P., Johnson, J. G., & Salzinger, S. (1998). A longitudinal analysis of risk factors for child maltreatment: Findings of a 17-year prospective study of officially recorded and self-reported child abuse and neglect. *Child Abuse and Neglect, 22*(11), 1065–1078.
Burks, V. S., Laird, R. D., Dodge, K. A., Pettit, G. S., & Bates, J. E. (1999). Knowledge structures, social information processing, and children's aggressive behavior. *Social Development, 8*(2), 220–236.
Currie, J., & Widom, C. S. (2010). Long-term consequences of child abuse and neglect on adult economic well-being. *Child Maltreatment, 15*(2), 111–120.
Crittenden, P. M. (1992). Children's strategies for coping with adverse home environments: An interpretation using attachment theory. *Child Abuse and Neglect, 16*(3), 329–343.
Dadds, M. R., Mullins, M. J., McAllister, R. A., & Atkinson, E. (2003). Attributions, affect, and behavior in abuse-risk mothers: A laboratory study. *Child Abuse and Neglect, 27*(1), 21–45.
Dixon, L., Browne, K., & Hamilton-Giachritsis, C. (2005a). Risk factors of parents abused as children: a mediational analysis of the intergenerational continuity of child maltreatment (Part I). *Journal of Child Psychology and Psychiatry, 46*(1), 47–57.
Dixon, L., Hamilton-Giachritsis, C., & Browne, K. (2005b). Attributions and behaviours of parents abused as children: A mediational analysis of the intergenerational continuity of child maltreatment (Part II). *Journal of Child Psychology and Psychiatry, 46*(1), 58–68.
Dodge, K. A., Bates, J. E., & Pettit, G. S. (1990). Mechanisms in the cycle of violence. *Science, 250*(4988), 1678–1683.
Dubowitz, H., Kim, J., Black, M. M., Weisbart, C., Semiatin, J., & Magder, L. S. (2011). Identifying children at high risk for a child maltreatment report. *Child Abuse & Neglect, 35*(2), 96–104.
Egeland, B., Jacobvitz, D., & Sroufe, L. A. (1988). Breaking the cycle of abuse. *Child Development* 1080–1088.
Frias-Armenta, M. (2002). Long-term effects of child punishment on Mexican women: A structural model. *Child Abuse and Neglect, 26*(4), 371–386.
Hildyard, K. L., & Wolfe, D. A. (2002). Child neglect: developmental issues and outcomes. *Child Abuse and Neglect, 26*(6), 679–695.
Institute of Medicine & National Research Council. (2014). *New directions in child abuse and neglect research*. Washington, DC: The National Academies Press
Jaffee, S. R., Bowes, L., Ouellet-Morin, I., Fisher, H. L., Moffitt, T. E., Merrick, M. T., et al. (2013). Safe, stable, nurturing relationships break the intergenerational cycle of abuse: A prospective nationally representative cohort of children in the United Kingdom. *Journal of Adolescent Health, 53*(4), S4–S10.
Kempe, C. H., Silverman, F. N., Steele, B. F., Droegemueller, W., & Silver, H. K. (1985). The battered-child syndrome. *Child Abuse and Neglect, 9*(2), 143–154.
Kim, K. (2012). The role of culture in theories of the intergenerational transmission of violence. *Child and Family Social Work, 17*, 395–405.
Kotchick, B. A., & Forehand, R. (2002). Putting parenting in perspective: A discussion of the contextual factors that shape parenting practices. *Journal of Child and Family Studies, 11*(3), 255–269.
Leve, L. D., Khurana, A., & Reich, E. B. (2015). Intergenerational transmission of maltreatment. A multilevel examination. *Development and Psychopathology, 27*, 1429–1442.
Li, F., Godinet, M. T., & Arnsberger, P. (2011). Protective factors among families with children at risk of maltreatment: Follow up to early school years. *Children and Youth Services Review, 33*(1), 139–148.
Lounds, J. J., Borkowski, J. G., & Whitman, T. L. (2006). The potential for child neglect: The case of adolescent mothers and their children. *Child Maltreatment, 11*(3), 281–294.

Marshall, J. M., Huang, H., & Ryan, J. P. (2011). Intergenerational families in child welfare: Assessing needs and estimating permanency. *Children and Youth Services Review, 33*(6), 1024–1030.
Milner, J. S. (1993). Social information processing and physical child abuse. *Clinical Psychology Review, 13*(3), 275–294.
Milner, J. S. (2003). Social information processing in high-risk and physically abusive parents. *Child Abuse and Neglect, 27*(1), 7–20.
Montes, M. P., de Paúl, J., & Milner, J. S. (2001). Evaluations, attributions, affect, and disciplinary choices in mothers at high and low risk for child physical abuse. *Child Abuse and Neglect, 25*(8), 1015–1036.
Pears, K. C., & Capaldi, D. M. (2001). Intergenerational transmission of abuse: a two-generational prospective study of an at-risk sample. *Child Abuse and Neglect, 25*(11), 1439–1461.
Price, J. M., & Landsverk, J. (1998). Social information-processing patterns as predictors of social adaptation and behavior problems among maltreated children in foster care. *Child Abuse and Neglect, 22*(9), 845–858.
Renner, L., & Slack, K. S. (2006). Intimate partner violence and child maltreatment: Understanding intra- and intergenerational connections. *Child Abuse & Neglect, 30*(6), 599–617.
Robboy, J., & Anderson, K. G. (2011). Intergenerational child abuse and coping. *Journal of Interpersonal Violence, 26*(17), 3526–3541.
Sidebotham, P. (2001). An ecological approach to child abuse: A creative use of scientific models in research and practice. *Child Abuse Review, 10*(2), 97–112.
Thompson, R. (2006). Exploring the link between maternal history of childhood victimization and child risk of maltreatment. *Journal of Trauma Practice, 5*(2), 57–72.
Thornberry, T. P., Henry, K. L., Smith, C. A., Ireland, T. O., Greenman, S. J., & Lee, R. D. (2013). Breaking the cycle of maltreatment: The role of safe, stable, and nurturing relationships. *Journal of Adolescent Health, 53*(4), S25–S31.
Valentino, K., Nutall, A. K., Comas, M., Borkowski, J. G., & Akai, C. E. (2012). Intergenerational continuity of child abuse among adolescent mothers: Authoritarian parenting, community violence, and race. *Child Maltreatment, 17*(2), 172–181.
Widom, C. S., & Wilson, H. W. (2015). Intergenerational transmission of violence. In J. Lindert & I. Levav (Eds.), *Violence and Mental Health* (pp. 27–45). Netherlands: Springer.
Zuravin, S., McMillen, C., DePanfilis, D., & Risley-Curtiss, C. (1996). The intergenerational cycle of child maltreatment continuity versus discontinuity. *Journal of Interpersonal Violence, 11*(3), 315–334.

Chapter 3
Summary of Research on Intergenerational Transmission of Child Maltreatment

3.1 Brief History of Research on Intergenerational Transmission of Child Maltreatment

The concept of intergenerational transmission of child maltreatment (ITCM) appeared in the earliest academic literature on child maltreatment.[1] In the seminal work of Kempe and colleagues (1962), which identified the battered child syndrome, the authors explain, "Beating of children, however is not confined to people with a psychopathic personality or of borderline socioeconomic status. It also occurs among people with good education and stable financial and social background… There is also some suggestion that the attacking parent was subjected to similar abuse in childhood." (p. 145). Kempe and colleagues (1962) continued explaining that this should be unsurprising considering that psychologists and social anthropologists have long understood that patterns of parenting are passed among generations and remain largely unchanged. Thus, in the article which is recognized as the identification of child maltreatment in medicine and the foundation of the understanding of child maltreatment, the concept of ITCM was present (Herzberger 1990).

The year after Kempe and colleagues' seminal work, Curtis (1963) published "*Violence breeds violence—perhaps?*" which outlined concerns that maltreated children would become "tomorrow's murderers and perpetrators of other crimes of violence if they survive" (p. 386). Curtis (1963) explained, "It is often pointed out that sadistic parents are likely to be repeating a pattern which they experienced with their own parents. How and why do these patterns originate? What factors influence them to wax and wane from one generation to the next? Under what circumstances does criminal violence overflow from the family into society?" (p. 387). Curtis was

[1]While our focus is on ITCM and parents who experienced abuse going on to abuse their children, the connection between child maltreatment and subsequent violence and criminal involvement was hypothesized and studied as earlier as the 1940s as is noted by Curtis (1963) who describes three studies from as early as 1940 that examine people who kill identified what we now call child maltreatment within the cases.

L. Schelbe and J.M. Geiger, *Intergenerational Transmission of Child Maltreatment*, SpringerBriefs in Social Work,
DOI 10.1007/978-3-319-43824-5_3

quick to point out that the consequences of child maltreatment are various and complicated and asserted "It is, of course, highly unlikely that there is any one-to-one relationship between child abuse and later crimes of violence" (p. 387). Throughout the 1960s and into the 1970s, multiple scholars and practitioners wrote that a parental history of maltreatment was one of the causes of child maltreatment (Spinetta and Rigler 1972).

In the 1980s, scholars called into question the wide acceptance of ITCM with Garbarino and Gilliam (1980) concluding that ITCM has not "passed scientific muster" (p. 111). Kaufman and Zigler (1987) reviewed the literature on ITCM and determined that, "The belief that abused children are likely to become abusive parents is widely accepted." Yet, asserted "its unqualified acceptance is unfounded" (p. 186). Widom (1989b) echoed her concern that the cycle of violence hypothesis is not inevitable and called for more empirical research using improved methods. During this time, there was an interest in designing methodologically sound studies to examine ITCM. Yet, many studies continued to have significant limitations.

While there were continued assertions that a parental history of maltreatment caused child maltreatment, the critique of ITCM continued in the 1990s. Herzberger (1990) examined ITCM research historically and called it "the cyclical hypothesis" since "The hypothesis was transformed into 'fact' as article after article cited it as though the hypothesis has been tested and confirmed" (p. 529). Herzberger (1990) included the early evidence used to support ITCM and explained, "Thus some of the lore about the strength of the evidence in favor of the cyclical hypothesis stems from inaccurate reading and reporting of the results of early studies" (p. 535). Herzberger (1990) asserted, "Today, we know that the cyclical hypothesis is overly simplistic and fails to tell much of the truth about the transmission of violence from one generation of a family to the next" (p. 529). A more complete discussion of the critiques of ITCM research appears in Chap. 6.

At the turn of the century, Ertem and colleagues (2000) developed methodological standards based upon a hypothetical experimental model of a randomized control trial to specifically study ITCM and, using these standards, evaluated 10 studies conducted between 1965 and 2000. Only one study met all eight criteria and one met six, and most studies failed to control for intervening factors. Ertem and colleagues (2000) note that only one study included a nationally representative sample and cautioned that as society changes, results from studies years ago may not be relevant later. Thus concluded, that even if studies all found support for ITCM—which they did not—more research would be needed.

Thornberry et al. (2012) updated Ertem and colleagues' (2000) study with refined methodological criteria and reviewed 47 articles. While most of the articles reviewed "report support for the cycle of maltreatment hypothesis," few of them met the basic methodological criteria (Thornberry et al. 2012, p. 144). Thornberry and colleagues (2012) determined that there existed only a rather modest relationship between history of maltreatment and perpetrating maltreatment or having a child who is maltreated and stated, "When the methodological rigor is taken into account, the level of support for the hypothesis becomes, in our view, much less certain" (p. 145). Thornberry and colleagues (2012) concluded, "We concur with

Ertem and colleagues' (2000) conclusion that there is likely to be significant association between maltreatment in the first generation and maltreatment in the second generation but, at the present time, there is insufficient scientific evidence to draw a definitive conclusion about the cycle of maltreatment hypothesis" (p. 145).

So how did the general acceptance of ITCM come to pass despite the fact that there is not a universal transmission? There are likely multiple contributing factors. As scholars have pointed out, ITCM makes intuitive sense as children learn from their parents (Garbarino and Gilliam 1980; Widom 1989a). The etiology of child maltreatment remains largely unknown, yet a parental history of maltreatment is a risk factor for child maltreatment. While there is no 100 % transmission rate, some parents who were maltreated as children do abuse and neglect their children. Thus, the acceptance of ITCM as a cause of maltreatment is likely due to the fact that parental history of child maltreatment is a risk factor. Practitioners may have embraced the idea of ITCM as they saw instances where parents who maltreated their children reported being maltreated. The number of scholarly publications about ITCM likely contributed to the acceptance of ITCM (Thornberry et al. 2012). Thornberry and colleagues (2012) explained that in their systematic review, they found 31 review articles which is almost as much as the 47 empirical articles in the systematic review, thus "the findings from a relatively small number, and in our view, methodologically weak number of studies appear to reverberate throughout the literature via a disproportionately large number of review articles, many of which do not evaluate the methodological rigor of the studies" (p. 146).

3.2 Overview of Research on Intergenerational Transmission of Child Maltreatment

The concept of ITCM is deceptively simple, the complexity becomes readily apparent when examining empirical studies about ITCM. One of the first places ITCM becomes complicated is when looking at outcomes—scholars sometime broadly use the term ITCM for outcomes rather than parental history of maltreatment impacting the maltreatment of their children. However, we are going to focus on ITCM in the most basic terms, taking a parental history of maltreatment impact on the next generation of child rearing. We are essentially examining the question to what extent does a parent's history of child maltreatment impact the parent maltreating his or her own children?

ITCM becomes complicated in how parental history of child maltreatment is defined and measured. Studies have relied on adults' retrospective accounts of child maltreatment, official records, or a combination of the two types of data, and as will be discussed in Chap. 6, there are important considerations with each data source. Also to complicate the matter more, there are multiple types of child maltreatment (e.g., neglect, physical abuse, emotional abuse, sexual abuse), and child maltreatment can vary greatly in chronicity and severity. This not only impacts how parental history of child maltreatment is conceptualized and measured, but also how child maltreatment in the next generation is understood. For example, Jaffee and colleagues (2013) found that mothers with a history of mild maltreatment (those who experienced one or two types of the five categories of maltreatment measured: emotional, physical, and sexual abuse, and emotional and physical neglect) were 3. 55 times more likely to have at least one child experience maltreatment by age 12 compared to mothers who did not have a history of maltreatment. They also found that mothers with a history of severe maltreatment (those who experienced at least three types of maltreatment) were 5.31 times more likely to have at least one child experience maltreatment by age 12 compared to mothers who did not have a history of maltreatment.

The way that data are interpreted in ITCM studies can also be problematic. Herzberger (1990) reminded us that we can interpret data in multiple ways and provide a concrete example using Straus' work, which reports an 18 % transmission rate of child maltreatment: "One (interpretation of the data) is that having been abused oneself leads to a 40 % increase in the likelihood that one will become an abuser, thus confirming the cyclical hypothesis. A second interpretation is that the cyclical hypothesis is wrong; over 80 % of adults who experience physical punishment in their youth did not abuse their own children." (p. 536). This example further illustrates that interpretations and presentation of findings should be viewed critically and with caution.

3.3 Empirical Studies on Intergenerational Transmission of Child Maltreatment

What do we actually know about ITCM? Despite the fact that scholars have been writing about and studying ITCM for several decades, we still definitively know little about ITCM. Despite the many methodological problems and mixed findings in ITCM research, reviews of ITCM research conclude ITCM likely exists (Ertem et al. 2000; Thornberry et al. 2012). Studies have found various transmission rates, as are noted in Table 3.1, that range from 4.99 to 54.3 % (e.g., Ben-David et al. 2015; Berlin et al. 2011; Dixon et al. 2009; Pears and Capaldi 2001; Valentino et al. 2012). This means that many parents who were maltreated will go on to maltreat their children; however, a parental history of maltreatment does not conclusively determine that parents will maltreat their children (e.g., Kaufman and Zigler 1987; Pears and Capaldi 2001; Sidebotham et al. 2001; Widom and Wilson 2015).

Although, we do not understand definitively what causes child maltreatment or ITCM, there are several factors identified that contribute to the continuity or discontinuity of ITCM. Studies have only started to examine what types of maltreatment and under what conditions ITCM occurs. As we discuss in Chaps. 4 and 5, there are multiple risk and protective factors that can contribute to ITCM. The reality is that while empirical studies have expanded our knowledge about ITCM, there are many more questions that need to be answered. See Chap. 6 for a discussion about future direction in research.

Table 3.1 Summary of key intergenerational transmission of child maltreatment studies

Author(s) (year)	Transmission rate[a]	Maltreatment type[b]	Factors[c]	Self-reports[d]	Official reports[e]
Altemeier et al. (1986)	N/A	P	Y	G1	G2
Ball (2009)	N/A	P	Y	G1	N
Banyard et al. (2003)	N/A	P/S	Y	G1	G1
Bartlett and Easterbrooks (2012)	44 %	P/N	N	G1	G2
Ben-David et al. (2015)	4.99 %	Multi	Y	N	G1, G2
Berlin et al. (2011)	16.7	P/N	Y	G1	G2
Coohey and Braun (1997)	N/A	P/N	Y	G1	G2
Conger et al. (2013)	N/A	Multi	Y	N	N[f]
Cort et al. (2011)	46.7 %	Multi	N	G1	G2
DiLillo et al. (2000)	N/A	P/S	Y	G1	N
Dixon et al. (2005a, b, 2009)	6.7 %	P/S	Y	G1	G2
Egeland et al. (1988)	N/A	Multi	Y	G1	N[f]
Finkelhor et al. (1997)	N/A	S	Y	G1	N
Folsom et al. (2003)	N/A	Multi	Y	N	G2[g]
Frias-Armenta (2002)	N/A	P	Y	G1	G1, G2
Haapasalo and Aaltonen (1999)	N/A	P/E	Y	G1, G2	G2
Herrenkohl et al. (2013)	N/A	P	Y	G1, G2	N
Heyman and Smith Slep (2002)	N/A	P	Y	G1, G2	N
Hunter and Kilstrom (1979)	18.36 %	Multi	Y	G1	G2
Jaffee et al. (2013)	46 %	P	Y	G1, G2	N
Lounds et al. (2006)	N/A	N	Y	G1	N
Newcomb and Locke (2001)	N/A	P/S/N/E	N	G1	N
Oates et al. (1998)	34 %	S	N	G1	G2
Pears and Capaldi (2001)	23 %	Multi	Y	G1	G2
Renner and Slack (2006)	N/A	P/S/N	Y	G1	G2
Sidebotham et al. (2001)	10–13 %	P/S/N/E	Y	G1	G2
Smith and Adler (1991)	N/A	Multi	Y	G1	N[h]
Straus (1979)	N/A	P	Y	G1	N

(continued)

Table 3.1 (continued)

Author(s) (year)	Transmission rate[a]	Maltreatment type[b]	Factors[c]	Self-reports[d]	Official reports[e]
Thompson (2006)	N/A	P/S	Y	G1	G2
Thornberry et al. (2013)	14.9 %	Multi	Y	N	G1, G2
Valentino et al. (2012)	54.3 %	P/S/E	Y	G1/G2	N
Widom (1989a)	N/A	P/S/N	N	N	G1, G2
Widom et al. (2015)	21.4 %	Multi	N	G1, G2	G1, G2
Wolock and Horowitz (1979)	N/A	Multi	Y	G1	G2
Zuravin et al. (1996)	N/A	P/S/N	N	G1	G2

This table summarizes rigorous studies of ITCM and highlights components of the studies
[a]Transmission rate of ITCM
[b]Maltreatment type P = physical abuse, S = sexual abuse, N = neglect, E = emotional or psychological abuse, Multi = multiple types of maltreatment examined together
[c]Risk, protective, or contextual factors were taken into consideration into the study; Y = yes and N = no
[d]Self-reports of maltreatment were used; G1 = parent's report of history of child maltreatment, G2 = child's report of child maltreatment, and N = no
[e]Official reports of maltreatment were used; G1 = official report of parent history of child maltreatment, G2 = official report of child's maltreatment, and N = no
[f]Maltreatment measured through observations of G1 and G2
[g]Case review for G1 identified maltreatment
[h]Hospital records identified maltreatment for G2

3.3.1 Key Studies

Table 3.1 summarizes the key studies that have examined ITCM. Once again, we offer the disclaimer that we are just focusing on ITCM and there are many other studies that have examined other forms of violence and other outcomes that are related to experiencing maltreatment as a child. This table is not exhaustive, rather, it focuses on the most rigorous studies and provides a broad overview of ITCM research.

Hunter and Kilstrom (1979) conducted one of the earliest studies to focus on ITCM specifically. They followed a small sample of families to determine maltreatment in the child's first year. Of the 49 families, 9 had a record of maltreatment after the first year. Later, researchers began examining variables associated with those who were able to break the cycle of violence in their families and those who were unable. Egeland and colleagues (1988) concluded that more than half of the mothers did go on to maltreat their children, and the authors identified several factors related to breaking the cycle among a small sample of mothers related to relationships, support, and resources. In the early to mid-2000s, several studies emerged examining the transmission of child maltreatment and violence. For example, Dixon and colleagues used a small community sample to examine maltreatment among families with a history of child maltreatment and found a small proportion of parents went on to maltreat their child within the first 13 months of their life. Pears and Capaldi (2001) used a two-generation sample from the Oregon Youth Study and found that parents who had experienced maltreatment as a child were slightly more than twice as likely to have children who reported being abused compared with those parents who had not experienced childhood maltreatment. As will be discussed in Chap. 7, many of these studies acknowledged a number of methodological limitations.

Widom (1989a, b; Widom et al. 2015) has published a number of studies that focus on whether there is an intergenerational transmission of violence in families and what mechanisms promote and inhibit this process. Her examination of ITCM through prospective cohort designs has found mixed support for ITCM, and she has cautioned that a parental history of child maltreatment does not translate to future generations of child maltreatment. Widom et al. (2015) conclude that ITCM is "more complex and challenging than expected" (p. 1484).

More recent studies have aimed to examine not only the transmission rate of child maltreatment across generations, but also the mediating and moderating variables that increase and decrease the risk of transmission. This helps us to understand better what the risk and protective factors are that can be used to inform interventions and supports targeting those who experience maltreatment. For example, Berlin and colleagues (2011) examined type of maltreatment and the factors that mediate the relationship in generational transmission. In a special issue of the Journal of Adolescent Health, the authors specifically focus on safe, stable, nurturing relationships (SSNRs) as variables that may interrupt the transmission of child maltreatment (Conger et al. 2013; Herrenkohl et al. 2013; Jaffee et al. 2013; Schofield et al. 2013; Thornberry et al. 2013).

Few qualitative studies of ITCM exist, however, they provide some valuable insights into understanding ITCM. For example, using interviews with parents identified by child protective services for being at risk for their children being removed from their care, McWey and colleagues (2013) identified a potential typology of ITCM based on patterns, beliefs, and behaviors. Most parents recognized the intergenerational pattern of maltreatment and said they wanted to be different, yet many parents described engaging in "destructive" parenting actions. Studies such as McWey and colleagues' (2013) have important implications for practice, and can also guide larger quantitative studies.

3.4 Conclusion

Beginning with the earliest academic literature on child maltreatment, scholars have discussed the hypothesis of ITCM. Over the last half century, studies have examined ITCM and found varying levels of support for the concept. There are limitations to the research on ITCM that stem from methodological considerations including operationalization of parental history of maltreatment, measurement of child maltreatment, sampling, and design. Dixon and colleagues (2005a) concluded that with the wide variation in rates due to methodological issues:

> Therefore, it is very difficult to make any overarching estimates about the proportion of parents with a history of child abuse that go onto maltreat their child, especially when cultural differences are taken into account. However, methodological issues alone cannot account for the fact that only a minority of parents with a history of childhood abuse go on to abuse their own children (p. 48).

As we will discuss in Chap. 6, there are many opportunities for future research to better understand ITCM.

References

Altemeier, W. A., O'Connor, S., Sherrod, K. B., Tucker, D., & Vietze, P. (1986). Outcome of abuse during childhood among pregnant low income women. *Child Abuse and Neglect, 10*(3), 319–330.

Ball, J. D. (2009). Intergenerational transmission of abuse of incarcerated fathers: A study of the measurement of abuse. *Journal of Family Issues, 30*(3), 371–390.

Banyard, V. L., Williams, L. M., & Siegel, J. A. (2003). The impact of complex trauma and depression on parenting: An exploration of mediating risk and protective factors. *Child Maltreatment, 8*(4), 334–349.

Bartlett, J., & Easterbrooks, M. (2012). Links between physical abuse in childhood and child neglect among adolescent mothers. *Children and Youth Services Review, 34*, 2164–2169.

Ben-David, V., Jonson-Reid, M., Drake, B., & Kohl, P. (2015). The association between childhood maltreatment experiences and the onset of maltreatment perpetration in young adulthood controlling for proximal and distal factors. *Child Abuse and Neglect, 46*, 132–141.

Berlin, L. J., Appleyard, K., & Dodge, K. A. (2011). Intergenerational continuity in child maltreatment: Mediating mechanisms and implications for prevention. *Child Development, 82* (1), 162–176.

Coohey, C., & Braun, N. (1997). Toward an integrated framework for understanding child physical abuse. *Child Abuse and Neglect, 21*(11), 1081–1094.

Conger, R. D., Schofield, T. J., Neppl, T. K., & Merrick, M. T. (2013). Disrupting intergenerational continuity in harsh and abusive parenting: The importance of a nurturing relationship with a romantic partner. *Journal of Adolescent Health, 53*(4), S11–S17.

Cort, N. A., Toth, S. L., Cerulli, C., & Rogosch, F. (2011). Maternal intergenerational transmission of childhood multitype maltreatment. *Journal of Aggression, Maltreatment & Trauma, 20*(1), 20–39.

Curtis, G. C. (1963). Violence breeds violence-perhaps? *American Journal of Psychiatry, 120*(4), 386–387.

DiLillo, D., Tremblay, G. C., & Peterson, L. (2000). Linking childhood sexual abuse and abusive parenting: The mediating role of maternal anger. *Child Abuse and Neglect, 24*(6), 767–779.

Dixon, L., Browne, K., & Hamilton-Giachritsis, C. (2005a). Risk factors of parents abused as children: a mediational analysis of the intergenerational continuity of child maltreatment (Part I). *Journal of Child Psychology and Psychiatry, 46*(1), 47–57.

Dixon, L., Hamilton-Giachritsis, C., & Browne, K. (2005b). Attributions and behaviours of parents abused as children: A mediational analysis of the intergenerational continuity of child maltreatment (Part II). *Journal of Child Psychology and Psychiatry, 46*(1), 58–68.

Dixon, L., Browne, K., & Hamilton-Giachritsis, C. (2009). Patterns of risk and protective factors in the intergenerational cycle of maltreatment. *Journal of Family Violence, 24*(2), 111–122.

Egeland, B., Jacobvitz, D., & Sroufe, L. A. (1988). Breaking the cycle of abuse. *Child Development*, 1080–1088.

Ertem, I. O., Leventhal, J. M., & Dobbs, S. (2000). Intergenerational continuity of child physical abuse: How good is the evidence? *The Lancet, 356*(9232), 814–819.

Finkelhor, D., Moore, D., Hamby, S. L., & Straus, M. A. (1997). Sexually abused children in a national survey of parents: Methodological issues. *Child Abuse and Neglect, 21*(1), 1–9.
Folsom, W. S., Christensen, M. L., Avery, L., & Moore, C. (2003). The co-occurrence of child abuse and domestic violence: An issue of service delivery for social service professionals. *Child and Adolescent Social Work Journal, 20*(5), 375–387.
Frias-Armenta, M. (2002). Long-term effects of child punishment on Mexican women: A structural model. *Child Abuse and Neglect, 26*(4), 371–386.
Garbarino, J., & Gilliam, G. (1980). *Understanding abusive families*. Lexington, MA: Lexington Books.
Haapasalo, J., & Aaltonen, T. (1999). Mothers' abusive childhood predicts child abuse. *Child Abuse Review, 8*(4), 231–250.
Herrenkohl, T. I., Klika, J. B., Brown, E. C., Herrenkohl, R. C., & Leeb, R. T. (2013). Tests of the mitigating effects of caring and supportive relationships in the study of abusive disciplining over two generations. *Journal of Adolescent Health, 53*(4), S18–S24.
Herzberger, S. D. (1990). The cyclical pattern of child abuse: A study of research methodology. *The American Behavioral Scientist, 33*(5), 529.
Heyman, R. E., & Smith Slep, A. M. (2002). Do child abuse and interparental violence lead to adulthood family violence? *Journal of Marriage and Family, 64*(4), 864–870.
Hunter, R. S., & Kilstrom, N. (1979). Breaking the cycle in abusive families. *The American Journal of Psychiatry, 136*(10), 1320–1322.
Jaffee, S. R., Bowes, L., Ouellet-Morin, I., Fisher, H. L., Moffitt, T. E., Merrick, M. T., et al. (2013). Safe, stable, nurturing relationships break the intergenerational cycle of abuse: A prospective nationally representative cohort of children in the United Kingdom. *Journal of Adolescent Health, 53*(4), S4–S10.
Kaufman, J., & Zigler, E. (1987). Do abused children become abusive parents? *American Journal of Orthopsychiatry, 57*(2), 186.
Kempe, C. H., Silverman, F. N., Steele, B. F., Droegemueller, W., & Silver, H. K. (1962). The battered-child syndrome. *Journal of the American Medical Association, 181*, 17–24.
Lounds, J. J., Borkowski, J. G., & Whitman, T. L. (2006). The potential for child neglect: The case of adolescent mothers and their children. *Child Maltreatment, 11*(3), 281–294.
McWey, L. M., Pazdera, A. L., Vennum, A., & Wojciak, A. S. (2013). Intergenerational patterns of maltreatment in families at risk for foster care. *Journal of Marital and Family Therapy, 39*(2), 133–147.
Newcomb, M. D., & Locke, T. F. (2001). Intergenerational cycle of maltreatment: A popular concept obscured by methodological limitations. *Child Abuse and Neglect, 25*(9), 1219–1240.
Oates, R. K., Tebbutt, J., Swanston, H., Lynch, D. L., & O'Toole, B. I. (1998). Prior childhood sexual abuse in mothers of sexually abused children. *Child Abuse and Neglect, 22*(11), 1113–1118.
Pears, K. C., & Capaldi, D. M. (2001). Intergenerational transmission of abuse: A two-generational prospective study of an at-risk sample. *Child Abuse and Neglect, 25*(11), 1439–1461.
Renner, L., & Slack, K. S. (2006). Intimate partner violence and child maltreatment: Understanding intra- and intergenerational connections. *Child Abuse and Neglect, 30*(6), 599–617.
Sidebotham, P., Golding, J., & ALSPAC Study Team. (2001). Child maltreatment in the "Children of the Nineties": A longitudinal study of parental risk factors. *Child Abuse and Neglect, 25*(9), 1177–1200.
Smith, J. A., & Adler, R. G. (1991). Children hospitalized with child abuse and neglect: A case-control study. *Child Abuse and Neglect, 15*, 437–445.
Spinetta, J. J., & Rigler, D. (1972). The child-abusing parent: A psychological review. *Psychological Bulletin, 77*(4), 296.
Straus, M. A. (1979). Family patterns and child abuse in a nationally representative American sample. *Child Abuse and Neglect, 3*(1), 213–225.

Thompson, R. (2006). Exploring the link between maternal history of childhood victimization and child risk of maltreatment. *Journal of Trauma Practice, 5*(2), 57–72.

Thornberry, T. P., Henry, K. L., Smith, C. A., Ireland, T. O., Greenman, S. J., & Lee, R. D. (2013). Breaking the cycle of maltreatment: The role of safe, stable, and nurturing relationships. *Journal of Adolescent Health, 53*(4), S25–S31.

Thornberry, T. P., Knight, K. E., & Lovegrove, P. J. (2012). Does maltreatment beget maltreatment? A systematic review of the intergenerational literature. *Trauma, Violence, & Abuse, 13*(3), 135–152.

Valentino, K., Nuttall, A., Comas, M., Borkowski, J., & Akai, C. (2012). Intergenerational continuity of child abuse among adolescent mothers: Authoritarian parenting, community violence, and race. *Child Maltreatment, 17*, 172–181.

Widom, C. S. (1989a). Child abuse, neglect, and adult behavior: research design and findings on criminality, violence, and child abuse. *American Journal of Orthopsychiatry, 59*(3), 355–367.

Widom, C. S. (1989b). Does violence beget violence? A critical examination of the literature. *Psychological Bulletin, 106*(1), 3–28.

Widom, C. S., Czaja, S. J., & DuMont, K. A. (2015). Intergenerational transmission of child abuse and neglect: Real or detection bias? *Science, 347*(6229), 1480–1485.

Widom, C. S., & Wilson, H. W. (2015). Intergenerational transmission of violence. In J. Lindert & I. Levav (Eds.), *Violence and mental health* (pp. 27–45). Netherlands: Springer.

Wolock, I., & Horowitz, B. (1979). Child maltreatment and material deprivation among AFDC-recipient families. *The Social Service Review*, 175–194.

Zuravin, S., McMillen, C., DePanfilis, D., & Risley-Curtiss, C. (1996). The intergenerational cycle of child maltreatment continuity versus discontinuity. *Journal of Interpersonal Violence, 11*(3), 315–334.

Chapter 4
Risk Factors Associated with Intergenerational Transmission of Child Maltreatment

4.1 Risk Factors Associated with Child Maltreatment and the Intergenerational Transmission of Child Maltreatment

Many individual characteristics, family circumstances, and environmental factors influence the occurrence of child maltreatment as well as the intergenerational transmission of child maltreatment (ITCM). Risk factors associated with child maltreatment and ITCM are best examined with an ecological perspective in order to capture factors related to the individual, the family, and their environment (Belsky 1993; Li et al. 2011; Kotch et al. 1999; Sidebotham et al. 2001; Zielinski and Bradshaw 2006). These risk factors, related to the parent, the child, and the family's environment, increase the likelihood of child maltreatment. Much of the research on the mediators of parental history of child maltreatment and the perpetration of child maltreatment with their own children involves examination of what is referred to as "cycle maintainers," those who go on to perpetuate maltreatment into the next generation. This chapter presents research regarding the risks for child maltreatment and the factors that have been shown to increase the risk for ITCM. It is important to note that over the last two decades studies conducted with varying sized samples, in different geographic areas and with diverse and homogenous samples, have come to mixed conclusions about the risk factors associated with ITCM.

L. Schelbe and J.M. Geiger, *Intergenerational Transmission of Child Maltreatment*, SpringerBriefs in Social Work,
DOI 10.1007/978-3-319-43824-5_4

4.2 Parent-Related Factors Associated with Child Maltreatment

Parental developmental and psychological resources are linked to parental functioning. For example, early childbearing and adolescent parenting have been identified as risk factors related to child abuse and neglect due the lack of educational attainment and social development that young parents typically lack (Dubowitz et al. 2011; Dukewich et al. 1996; Mersky et al. 2009; Sidebotham et al. 2001). In addition, young parents may not have appropriate expectations of the child's capabilities or may have skewed beliefs about child development and appropriate discipline. Maternal depression and psychiatric illness have also been associated with neglect and poor child outcomes (Dubowitz et al. 2011; Sidebotham et al. 2001).

A lack of parental empathy plays a role in the occurrence of child abuse and neglect (Bavolek 2000; Wiehe 1997). Many empathy related behaviors such as understanding, responsiveness, and unconditional positive regard are critical to healthy, successful parenting (De Paul and Guibert 2008; de Paúl et al. 2008; Hoffman 2000; Moor and Silvern 2006; Wiehe 1997). Caregivers who model empathy by demonstrating attentiveness and attunement to their child's needs, as well as displaying positive affective response during infancy and early childhood help create secure attachment (De Paul and Guibert 2008; Goleman 1995; Tempel 2007; Wiehe 1997). Research suggests that abusive parents tend to have lower displays of empathy compared with non-abusive parents, and child abuse tends to occur when parents lack empathy or they are unable to read the needs of their children accurately or to react in an appropriate way (Bavolek 2000; De Paul and Guibert 2008; de Paúl et al. 2008; Kilpatrick 2005; Wiehe 1997). Moor and Silvern (2006) found that child abuse and deficient parental empathy were strongly related to future psychological symptoms. Additionally, Tempel (2007) and Wiehe (1997) attribute the lack of empathy in abusive parents to exposure to significant stress in their home or community of origin and the lack of a positive model for empathic behavior.

Education level influences the occurrence of child maltreatment. In general, studies have shown that parents who graduate from high school (mostly mothers) are less likely to be reported for maltreatment (Budd et al. 2000; Kotch et al. 1999; Li et al. 2011; Sidebotham et al. 2001). Education achievement can influence income levels, health, and levels of unemployment (Baum et al. 2010) and can equate to better resources and housing. On the other hand, the lack of education can limit employment opportunities, income, and child care options, having a marked influence on the potential for child maltreatment. Among a group of adolescent mothers, Dukewich and colleagues (1996) found that among several factors, preparation for parenting (including knowledge and attitudes about children's development) was the strongest predictor of the potential for abuse.

Knowledge about parenting and child development has also been shown to be related to parental attitudes and practices. Having knowledge about developmental norms allows a parent to anticipate developmental changes in children and have appropriate expectations related to a child's age and development. Studies have shown that mothers with greater knowledge of infant and child development have more sophisticated parenting skills (Dukewich et al. 1996; Goodnow 1988; Huang et al. 2005). In general, greater parental knowledge is associated with more positive child developmental outcomes and greater parental competence. In addition, greater parental knowledge is related to higher socioeconomic status, income, and education levels (Conrad et al. 1992; Hess et al. 2004; Huang et al. 2005). An increase in knowledge about child development has been associated with a higher quality home environment and a lower risk of child maltreatment. Parents with an increased knowledge of child development tend to be more physically and verbally engaging and utilize fewer punitive discipline strategies (Dukewich et al. 1996; Huang et al. 2005). Parents' inaccurate beliefs or overestimation of their child's performance can actually undermine the child's performance (Belsky 1993).

Research shows that parental age (young parents) is associated with increased risk of child maltreatment (e.g., Bartlett and Easterbrooks 2012; Smith and Adler 1991; Stevens-Simon et al. 2001; Whitson et al. 2011). Studies show that adolescent mothers, in general, are more likely to exhibit abusive or neglectful parenting behaviors (Stevens-Simon et al. 2001; Whitson et al. 2011). It is postulated that younger parents may lack the cognitive functioning that helps to identify and meet the needs of their children or perhaps that younger parents do not have knowledge about appropriate child development (Bavolek and Keene 1999). Young parents typically have less income, are more likely to be unemployed, and have fewer established social supports (Afifi 2007; Lee and Goerge 1999). They are also less likely to be married and are more likely to be exposed to poverty (Lee and Goerge 1999).

Substance abuse and mental health issues can also contribute to an increased risk of child maltreatment. Parental substance abuse has been associated with higher rates of child neglect, in particular. Some estimate that substance abuse is co-occurring in up to 70 % of cases of child maltreatment (e.g., Brown and Anderson 1991; Locke and Newcomb 2003), and child welfare workers point to substance abuse as one of the biggest concerns facing child welfare (Daro and McCurdy 1992). Parental mental health issues can also contribute to child maltreatment. Mental illness is associated with heightened risk of child maltreatment. Parents who experience depression, schizophrenia, antisocial behaviors, and other undefined mental illness may exhibit less sensitivity to their child's needs, lower parenting quality, and greater disengagement (Chaffin et al. 1996; Kotch et al. 1999, Sheppard 1997; Walsh et al. 2002).

4.3 Parent-Related Factors Associated with Increased Risk for Intergenerational Transmission of Child Maltreatment

Several factors related to the parent have been shown to increase the potential for the intergenerational transmission of child maltreatment, including parental mental health, substance abuse, age, education, and relationships.

4.3.1 Early Parenting

In addition to being associated with increased risk of child maltreatment, parental age has also been linked to ITCM (Brown et al. 1998; Connelly and Straus 1992; Egeland and Brunnquell 1979; Lee 2009; Lee and Guterman 2010; Leventhal et al. 1984; Lynch and Roberts 1977; Kinard and Klerman 1980; Smith and Adler 1991). Among parents who have experienced child maltreatment, parental age when their first child was born has been shown to increase risk for the intergenerational transmission of child maltreatment. For example, Dixon and colleagues (2005) found parental age at first born child was one of the most significant risk factors for continuity of child abuse with maternal age inversely related to risk for child abuse. In another study on ITCM, Valentino and colleagues (2012) found 54.3 % continuity of child maltreatment among study subjects who were all adolescent parents. In a study conducted by Bartlett and Easterbrooks (2012) with young adolescent mothers (under age 17), mothers with a history of physical abuse in childhood were four times more likely to neglect their child than a young mother without a history of physical abuse. Similarly, Sidebotham and colleagues (2006), along with other risk factors, found that young parents with a history of child maltreatment were more likely to be investigated for child maltreatment or to have a child placed on the child protection register than those without a history of maltreatment.

Despite the dearth of literature regarding the causes or indicators of the increased risk of ITCM among young parents, it is believed that young parental age has been identified as a risk factor for child maltreatment because it is associated with a lack of resources, experience, and knowledge about parenting. Young parents may be less mature, responsible, and focused on themselves instead of a child in their care, which may contribute to the contextual factors associated with child maltreatment, particularly neglect. Several factors have been identified as indicators of early childbearing that are also associated with child maltreatment, such as low socioeconomic status, a history of child maltreatment, and stress (Lee and Goerge 1999).

4.3.2 Parental Mental Health

Parental mental health problems has also been shown to be a mediator of the association between parental experience of child maltreatment and their child's own experience of child abuse or neglect. For example, in their large prospective cohort study, Sidebotham and colleagues (2006) found that a psychiatric history increased the risk of ITCM by over 2.5 times that of the baseline population. Several studies confirmed that depressive symptoms linked a history of child maltreatment and perpetrating child maltreatment (Dixon et al. 2005a, 2005b; Frias-Armenta 2002; Pears and Capaldi 2001; Thompson 2006). Jaffee and colleagues (2013) found that mothers with a history of child maltreatment were more likely to have mental health problems, and those in their sample deemed "cycle maintainers" experienced more depression and antisocial behavior. However, several studies did not find depression or other mental health problems to mediate the relationship between history of child maltreatment and ITCM (Berlin et al. 2011; Cort et al. 2011). Although mental health problems have been shown to increase the risk for ITCM, the experience of maltreatment as a child may cause or exacerbate symptoms of mental illness for the parent. A history of trauma can also impact the incidence of ITCM (Banyard et al. 2003; Belsky et al. 2009; Berlin et al. 2011; Neppl et al. 2009).

4.3.3 Substance Abuse

The presence of a parental substance abuse problem can create an unstable family environment, stress, and the potential for child maltreatment. Adults who have experienced child maltreatment and other adverse childhood experiences are at risk of developing substance abuse disorders (e.g., Anda et al. 2006; MacMillan et al. 2001; Widom et al. 2007), and parental substance abuse has been associated with child maltreatment (e.g., Chaffin et al. 1996). Several studies point to substance abuse problems as a factor that increases the risk of child maltreatment among parents who have experienced maltreatment themselves (Appleyard et al. 2011; Dixon et al. 2009; Frias-Armenta 2002; Jaffee et al. 2013; Kotch et al. 1999).

4.3.4 Other Parent-Related Factors Related to Intergenerational Transmission of Child Maltreatment

Other factors, such as parent's level of education (Ben-David et al. 2015; Sidebotham et al. 2001, 2006), history of adolescent delinquency (Thornberry et al. 2003), type of child maltreatment experienced by the parent (Cort et al. 2011;

Dilillo and Damashek 2003), and partner choice (Leve et al. 2015) have also been examined as mediators in a parent's history of child maltreatment and the intergenerational continuity or transmission of child maltreatment.

Some studies have shown that parents with a history of adolescent delinquency, and who have experienced maltreatment as a child, are at greater risk of maltreatment with their own children (Thornberry et al. 2003). Researchers point to a possible predisposition to violence or antisocial behavior that leads to both delinquency and child maltreatment perpetration as well as the inability to form positive interpersonal relationships, which is common among individuals who have experienced maltreatment.

Research has explored the type of maltreatment experienced by the parent as an indicator of ITCM as well as the risks associated with the type of maltreatment perpetrated by parents who have experienced child maltreatment. For example, Cort and colleagues (2011) examined multitype maltreatment among two generations and found that a mother's experience of multiple types of maltreatment predicted a child's experience of multitype maltreatment. Dilillo and Damashek (2003) conducted a study with mothers who had experienced child sexual abuse and found that many child sexual abuse survivors in their sample experienced difficulties with some aspects of parenting, such as setting clear boundaries. They also found that they may be more likely to use harsh physical discipline with their own children.

4.4 Child-Related Factors Associated with Increased Risk for Child Maltreatment

The interaction between caregiver and child and factors related to the child, such as the child's disposition, special needs, and personality can also influence parental attitudes and behaviors. There is indication in the literature suggesting that the child's age, physical health and/or behavior can be predictive of child maltreatment. For example, younger children are more dependent on their caregivers and more physically vulnerable to injury due to developmental reasons, such as the inability to walk and/or speak (Belsky 1993). Young children also have a harder time expressing themselves verbally and are less able to regulate their emotions, requiring greater capacity for parents to interpret the needs of their children accurately. Children with disabilities, developmental delays, cognitive impairment, or failure to thrive may be at increased risk for maltreatment (Dubowitz et al. 2011; Hibbard and Desch 2007; Skuse et al. 1995). A child's temperament, mental health and behavioral needs have also been shown to influence parenting orientation (Putnam et al. 2002).

4.5 Child-Related Factors Associated with Increased Risk for Intergenerational Transmission of Child Maltreatment

Research has been conducted on the incidence of ITCM and developmental stage, as this can impact the child's behavior, abilities, and reactivity. Thornberry and Henry (2013) examined the timing of maltreatment and the subsequent risk of ITCM among a group of youth in New York. They found that maltreatment during adolescence significantly increases the odds of perpetrating child maltreatment as an adult when compared to children who had been maltreated earlier in their childhood. A study by Scarmella and Conger (2003) examined three generations for links in child maltreatment, parental behavior, and child's behavior. They hypothesized that a child's behavior problems would influence child maltreatment and found that hostile parenting in the second generation was positively related to problem behaviors among children in the next (third) generation. However, the continuity of hostile parenting in the third generation occurred only when those children were rated as highly reactive and emotionally negative. Hunter and colleagues (1978) studied newborns in an intensive care unit and found that children were more likely to be maltreated upon discharge when there was a family history of child maltreatment. They concluded that children's individual characteristics likely contributed to determining which of the vulnerable parents maltreated their children.

4.6 Family Factors Associated with Increased Risk for Child Maltreatment

Social isolation can be characterized as having the lack of a social support network, which includes tangible and emotional supports, access to information, programs, and positive social support from others. When parents and families are socially isolated, stress and a lack of resources creates increased risk for child maltreatment and neglect (Coohey and Braun 1997; Kelley et al. 1992). Social capital and cohesion is also influenced by one's community in how it supports parents and families with programs, accessibility, resources, and connection to people (Runyan et al. 1998). Social support has been shown to reduce the incidence of child maltreatment and is often included as a key element in child abuse prevention efforts with parents and families. When social support is not available to parents and other risks for child maltreatment exist, the likelihood for child abuse and/or neglect increases. Social support includes healthy relationships with family, partners, spouses, friends, and other parents. (Further discussion of social support as a protective factor against child maltreatment and ITCM is included in Chap. 5.) Emotional and tangible support can be helpful in reducing familial stress and therefore, child maltreatment.

It is fair to say that most times "when you know better, you do better" in that the cycle of maltreatment can be broken when parents are educated and have more knowledge about parenting, developmental expectations, services and programs, and appropriate discipline. (Education as a protective factor is also discussed further in Chap. 5 and as an intervention and as a prevention strategy in Chap. 7.)

4.7 Family Factors Associated with Increased Risk for Intergenerational Transmission of Child Maltreatment

4.7.1 Parenting and Family Environment

Social isolation is a risk factor for ITCM, although ITCM research has often examined the lack of social isolation and focused on the protective factor of social support. Detailed information about social support as a protective factor appears in Chap. 5. Berlin and colleagues (2011) examined social isolation as a mediator of ITCM and found that social isolation partially explained the association between mothers' childhood physical abuse and their children's maltreatment. Social support from family, friends, and others has been found central to reducing child maltreatment and ITCM (e.g., Dixon et al. 2009; Institute of Medicine and National Research Council 2014).

Parenting abilities, as well as parenting attitudes and practices, can influence ITCM. Several factors can impact how one views parenting and parenting skills among individuals who have experienced maltreatment. Individuals who have experienced maltreatment as a child can have varying life experiences following maltreatment. These individuals may also have experienced varying models of parenting—positive and negative. As a result, they can go on to perpetuate or choose not to continue dysfunctional parenting with their own children.

Parents' marital status and parenting styles have also been examined as mediating factors in ITCM. In general, single parents are more likely to report harsh parenting or physical discipline than parents in two-parent families (Brown et al. 1998) and may be at risk for lower quality caregiving than mother–father headed homes (Berger 2004). Dixon and colleagues (2005b) found that among parents who had experienced child maltreatment, parents who had negative attributions of the child, unrealistic perceptions of the child, poor caregiving quality, and poor parenting styles were at a greater risk of continuing the cycle of child maltreatment with their own children. Valentino and colleagues (2012) found that low levels of maternal authoritarian parenting attitudes were associated with the continuity of maltreatment. More consistent discipline was also found to be associated with less abuse by parents with a history of child abuse (Pears and Capaldi 2001).

4.7.2 Intimate Partner Violence

The family environment, whether healthy or unhealthy, can also increase the risk for child maltreatment, particularly among those who were previously in homes where there was violence, poor parenting or caregiving, neglect, or stress. One of the most studied factors affecting parents who also experienced child maltreatment is the presence of intimate partner violence and how it is manifested in parenting and how it co-occurs with ITCM and the family environment. Intimate partner violence is a complex phenomenon that often co-occurs with child maltreatment. The debate continues as to whether a child being present in a home where intimate partner violence occurs or witnessing intimate partner violence against one parent by another constitutes child maltreatment. There is no doubt, however, that violence in the home can have a significant impact on the family, the children, and those engaged in the violence.

Recent research has begun to address the co-occurrence of intimate partner violence and child maltreatment, the experience of maltreatment as a child and subsequently being a victim or perpetrator of intimate partner violence (Appel and Holden 1998; Moffitt and Caspi 2003; Dong et al. 2003; Renner and Slack 2006; Widom et al. 2014). In Appel and Holden's (1998) meta-analytic review, there was a rate of co-occurrence or overlap of almost 40 % of intimate partner violence and child maltreatment. Further, Folsom and colleagues (2003) reviewed files from 537 families at one agency (of which half were involved with child protective services) and found that almost half (48.9 %) experienced both child maltreatment and intimate partner violence and that two thirds of the sample had experienced childhood maltreatment and were experiencing issues of child maltreatment with their own children. Research also has shown that children exposed to violence in the home are at increased risk of relational violence during adolescence and adulthood (Heyman and Smith Slep 2002; Renner and Slack 2006; Smith et al. 2011), which could increase the risk of ITCM.

4.8 Contextual Factors Associated with Increased Risk for Child Maltreatment

In addition to parent and child related factors, various contextual factors such as potential sources of stress, support, socioeconomic status, and neighborhood have been shown to influence parenting attitudes and practices (Kotchick and Forehand 2002). Children may become at risk of child abuse and neglect when the child's needs are not being met by a parent or caregiver as a result of a lack of knowledge, resources, or because motivation or environmental and social supports are inadequate. Poverty and a lack of financial resources have been linked to the incidence of child abuse and neglect (Egeland et al. 1988) as well as several socioeconomic characteristics of neighborhoods and communities (Coulton et al. 2007; Drake and

Pandey 1996). The relationship between community level factors and child maltreatment is not surprising given that the risk of maltreatment is highly correlated with individual characteristics such as low socioeconomic status and education (Kim and Maguire-Jack 2015; Maguire-Jack 2014). Parents who struggle financially tend to have poorer living conditions and health issues that are not addressed and which tend to interfere with optimal parenting. Parents living in substandard housing or experiencing financial problems may have difficulty meeting their children's basic needs (e.g., housing/shelter, food, and clothing) and may experience more housing instability and frequent moves. The emotional stress of lacking financial resources can compound an already tense and volatile environment and increase the risk of ITCM among subsequent generations.

4.9 Contextual Factors Associated with Increased Risk for Intergenerational Transmission of Child Maltreatment

Few studies have successfully isolated specific contextual factor variables related to child maltreatment or how these factors mediate childhood experiences of child maltreatment and ITCM. Lynch and Cicchetti (2002) examined the relationship between community violence and the family system and determined that children who had experienced violence reported more separation anxiety and less of a connection with their caregiver, which could impact their risk for ITCM. Straus (1979) concluded the "structure of the American family" as well as "the economic and psychological stress created by poverty and an unstable economic system" contribute to the continuation of child maltreatment (p. 224). While stressing maltreatment is not inevitable, the context influences child maltreatment.

Contextual and systemic factors, such as child welfare system and foster care involvement, can also play a role in the incidence of ITCM. Recent studies have begun to examine the parenting abilities, experiences, and child welfare involvement of parents who experienced child welfare system involvement and often maltreatment as a child. Ben-David and colleagues (2015) found spending time in foster care during adolescence was associated with continuing ITCM. Although very little research points to a direct relationship, the risk for child welfare system involvement is increased for the parents aging out of foster care (Dworsky 2015) and the challenges described by the parents in some studies points to an increased risk for child maltreatment (Aparicio et al. 2015, 2016; Radey et al. 2016). In studies examining the parenting experiences of youth who have aged out of foster care or who have experienced foster care discuss their fear of system involvement and their desire to be a "different" parent than theirs were and to break the cycle of maltreatment. These parents may also be more likely to be targeted, investigated, and therefore involved in the system as a result of their involvement in the child welfare system as children and youth (Widom et al. 2015).

4.10 Conclusion

In the last several decades, research has sought to identify individual, familial, and contextual factors that lead to child maltreatment. Many of the identified risk factors are related and co-occur, yet much of the research has examined specific risk factors in isolation rather than looking at the complex interaction of multiple risk factors (Institute of Medicine and National Resource Council 2014). There is some evidence that having multiple risk factors significantly increases the risk of child maltreatment (Brown et al. 1998) and ITCM (Dixon et al. 2005a).

Knowledge about risk factors has helped to develop programs to support parents and families who are at risk of various forms of maltreatment and family violence. It has also led to research examining the factors that increase the risk for ITCM among parents who have experienced childhood maltreatment. What is known about these risk factors is limited and there is still much to be learned about the groups of individuals and families who are at greater risk of ITCM.

References

Afifi, T. O. (2007). Child abuse and adolescent parenting: Developing a theoretical model from an ecological perspective. *Journal of Aggression, Maltreatment, and Trauma, 14*(3), 89–105.

Appleyard, K., Berlin, L. J., Rosanbalm, K. D., & Dodge, K. A. (2011). Preventing early child maltreatment: Implications from a longitudinal study of maternal abuse history, substance use problems, and offspring victimization. *Prevention Science, 12*, 139e49.

Anda, R. F., Felitti, V. J., Bremner, J. D., Walker, J. D., Whitfield, C. H., Perry, B. D., et al. (2006). The enduring effects of abuse and related adverse experiences in childhood. *European Archives of Psychiatry and Clinical Neuroscience, 256*(3), 174–186.

Aparicio, E. M., Gioia, D., & Pecukonis, E. V. (2016). "I can get through this and I will get through this": The unfolding journey of teenage motherhood in and beyond foster care. *Qualitative Social Work.*

Aparicio, E., Pecukonis, E. V., & O'Neale, S. (2015). "The love that I was missing": Exploring the lived experience of motherhood among teen mothers in foster care. *Children and Youth Services Review, 51*, 44–54.

Appel, A. E., & Holden, G. W. (1998). The co-occurrence of spouse and physical child abuse: A review and appraisal. *Journal of Family Psychology, 12*(4), 578.

Baum, S., Ma, J., & Payea, K. (2010). *Education Pays, 2010: The benefits of higher education for individuals and society*. Trends in Higher Education Series: College Board Advocacy & Policy Center.

Bartlett, J., & Easterbrooks, M. (2012). Links between physical abuse in childhood and child neglect among adolescent mothers. *Children and Youth Services Review, 34*, 2164–2169.

Banyard, V. L., Williams, L. M., & Siegel, J. A. (2003). The impact of complex trauma and depression on parenting: An exploration of mediating risk and protective factors. *Child maltreatment, 8*(4), 334–349.

Bavolek, S. J. (2000). *The Nurturing Parenting Programs*. Washington, DC: Office of Juvenile Justice and Delinquency Prevention.

Bavolek, S. J., & Keene, R. G. (1999). *Adult-Adolescent Parenting Inventory (AAPI-2) administration and development handbook*. Park City, UT: Family Development Resources Inc.

Belsky, J. (1993). Etiology of child maltreatment: A developmental-ecological analysis. *Psychological Bulletin, 114*(3), 413–434.

Belsky, J., Conger, R., & Capaldi, D. M. (2009). The intergenerational transmission of parenting: Introduction to the special section. *Developmental Psychology, 45*(5), 1201.

Ben-David, V., Jonson-Reid, M., Drake, B., & Kohl, P. (2015). The association between childhood maltreatment experiences and the onset of maltreatment perpetration in young adulthood controlling for proximal and distal factors. *Child Abuse and Neglect, 46*, 132–141.

Berger, L. M. (2004). Income, family structure, and child maltreatment risk. *Children and Youth Services Review, 26*(8), 725–748.

Berlin, L. J., Appleyard, K., & Dodge, K. A. (2011). Intergenerational continuity in child maltreatment: Mediating mechanisms and implications for prevention. *Child Development, 82*(1), 162–176.

Brown, G. R., & Anderson, B. (1991). Psychiatric morbidity in adult inpatients with childhood histories of sexual and physical abuse. *American Journal of Psychiatry, 148*, 55–61.

Brown, J., Cohen, P., Johnson, J. G., & Salzinger, S. (1998). A longitudinal analysis of risk factors for child maltreatment: Findings of a 17-year prospective study of officially recorded and self-reported child abuse and neglect. *Child Abuse and Neglect, 22*(11), 1065–1078.

Budd, K. S., Heilman, N. E., & Kane, D. (2000). Psychosocial correlates of child abuse potential in multiply disadvantaged adolescent mothers. *Child Abuse and Neglect, 24*(5), 611–625.

Chaffin, M., Kelleher, K., & Hollenberg, J. (1996). Onset of physical abuse and neglect: Psychiatric, substance abuse, and social risk factors from prospective community data. *Child Abuse and Neglect, 20*(3), 191–203.

Connelly, C. D., & Straus, M. A. (1992). Mother's age and risk for physical abuse. *Child Abuse and Neglect, 16*(5), 709–718.

Conrad, B., Gross, D., Fogg, L., & Ruchala, P. (1992). Maternal confidence, knowledge, and quality of mother-toddler interactions: a preliminary study. *Infant Mental Health Journal, 13*(4), 353–362.

Coohey, C., & Braun, N. (1997). Toward an integrated framework for understanding child physical abuse. *Child Abuse and Neglect, 21*(11), 1081–1094.

Cort, N. A., Toth, S. L., Cerulli, C., & Rogosch, F. (2011). Maternal intergenerational transmission of childhood multitype maltreatment. *Journal of Aggression, Maltreatment & Trauma, 20*(1), 20–39.

Coulton, C. J., Crampton, D. S., Irwin, M., Spilsbury, J. C., & Korbin, J. E. (2007). How neighborhoods influence child maltreatment: A review of the literature and alternative pathways. *Child Abuse and Neglect, 31*(11), 1117–1142.

Daro, D., & McCurdy, K. (1992). Current trends in child abuse reporting and fatalities: The results of the 1991 annual fifty state survey. Working paper #808 (pp. 1–24). Chicago, IL7: National Committee for the Prevention of Child Abuse.

DiLillo, D., & Damashek, A. (2003). Parenting characteristics of women reporting a history of childhood sexual abuse. *Child Maltreatment, 8*(4), 319–333.

Dixon, L., Browne, K., & Hamilton-Giachritsis, C. (2005a). Risk factors of parents abused as children: a mediational analysis of the intergenerational continuity of child maltreatment (Part I). *Journal of Child Psychology and Psychiatry, 46*(1), 47–57.

Dixon, L., Hamilton-Giachritsis, C., & Browne, K. (2005b). Attributions and behaviours of parents abused as children: A mediational analysis of the intergenerational continuity of child maltreatment (Part II). *Journal of Child Psychology and Psychiatry, 46*(1), 58–68.

Dixon, L., Browne, K., & Hamilton-Giachritsis, C. (2009). Patterns of risk and protective factors in the intergenerational cycle of maltreatment. *Journal of Family Violence, 24*(2), 111–122.

De Paul, J., & Guibert, M. (2008). Empathy and child neglect: A theoretical model. *Child Abuse and Neglect, 32*(11), 1063–1071.

de Paúl, J., Pérez-Albéniz, A., Guibert, M., Asla, N., & Ormaechea, A. (2008). Dispositional empathy in neglectful mothers and mothers at high risk for child physical abuse. *Journal of Interpersonal Violence, 23*(5), 670–684.

Dong, M., Anda, R. F., Dube, S. R., Giles, W. H., & Felitti, V. J. (2003). The relationship of exposure to childhood sexual abuse to other forms of abuse, neglect, and household dysfunction during childhood. *Child Abuse and Neglect, 27*(6), 625–639.

Drake, B., & Pandey, S. (1996). Understanding the relationship between neighborhood poverty and specific types of child maltreatment. *Child Abuse and Neglect, 20*(11), 1003–1018.
Dubowitz, H., Kim, J., Black, M. M., Weisbart, C., Semiatin, J., & Magder, L. S. (2011). Identifying children at high risk for a child maltreatment report. *Child Abuse and Neglect, 35*(2), 96–104.
Dukewich, T. L., Borkowski, J. G., & Whitman, T. L. (1996). Adolescent mothers and child abuse potential: An evaluation of risk factors. *Child Abuse and Neglect, 20*(11), 1031–1047.
Dworsky, A. (2015). Child welfare services involvement among the children of young parents in foster care. *Child Abuse and Neglect, 45*, 68–79.
Egeland, B., & Brunnquell, D. (1979). An at-risk approach to the study of child abuse: Some preliminary findings. *Journal of the American Academy of Child Psychiatry, 18*(2), 219–235.
Egeland, B., Jacobvitz, D., & Sroufe, L. A. (1988). Breaking the cycle of abuse. *Child Development,* 59 (4), 1080–1088.
Folsom, W. S., Christensen, M. L., Avery, L., & Moore, C. (2003). The co-occurrence of child abuse and domestic violence: An issue of service delivery for social service professionals. *Child and Adolescent Social Work Journal, 20*(5), 375–387.
Frias-Armenta, M. (2002). Long-term effects of child punishment on Mexican women: A structural model. *Child Abuse and Neglect, 26*(4), 371–386.
Goleman, D. (1995). *Emotional intelligence*. New York: Bantam.
Goodnow, J. J. (1988). Parents' ideas, actions, and feelings: Models and methods from developmental and social psychology. *Child Development, 59*, 286–320.
Hibbard, R. A., & Desch, L. W. (2007). Maltreatment of children with disabilities. *Pediatrics, 119*(5), 1018–1025.
Hess, C. R., Teti, D. M., & Hussey-Gardner, B. (2004). Self-efficacy and parenting of high-risk infants: The moderating role of parent knowledge of infant development. *Journal of Applied Developmental Psychology, 25*(4), 423–437.
Heyman, R. E., & Smith Slep, A. M. (2002). Do child abuse and interparental violence lead to adulthood family violence? *Journal of Marriage and Family, 64*(4), 864–870.
Hoffman, M. L. (2000). *Empathy and moral development: Implications for caring and justice.* New York: Cambridge University Press.
Huang, K. Y., Caughy, M. O. B., Genevro, J. L., & Miller, T. L. (2005). Maternal knowledge of child development and quality of parenting among White, African-American and Hispanic mothers. *Journal of Applied Developmental Psychology, 26*(2), 149–170.
Hunter, R. S., Kilstrom, N., Kraybill, E. N., & Loda, F. (1978). Antecedents of child abuse and neglect in premature infants: A prospective study in a newborn intensive care unit. *Pediatrics, 61*(4), 629.
Institute of Medicine and National Research Council. (2014). *New directions in child abuse and neglect research.* Washington, DC: The National Academies Press.
Jaffee, S. R., Bowes, L., Ouellet-Morin, I., Fisher, H. L., Moffitt, T. E., Merrick, M. T., et al. (2013). Safe, stable, nurturing relationships break the intergenerational cycle of abuse: A prospective nationally representative cohort of children in the United Kingdom. *Journal of Adolescent Health, 53*(4), S4–S10.
Kelley, M. L., Power, T. G., & Wimbush, D. D. (1992). Determinants of Disciplinary Practices in Low-Income Black Mothers. *Child Development, 63*(3), 573–582.
Kilpatrick, K. L. (2005). The parental empathy measure: a new approach to assessing child maltreatment risk. *American Journal of Orthopsychiatry, 75*(4), 608.
Kim, B., & Maguire-Jack, K. (2015). Community interaction and child maltreatment. *Child Abuse and Neglect, 41*, 146–157.
Kinard, E., & Klerman, L. V. (1980). Teenage parenting and child abuse: Are they related? *American Journal of Orthopsychiatry, 50*(3), 481.
Kotch, J. B., Browne, D. C., Dufort, V., Winsor, J., & Catellier, D. (1999). Predicting child maltreatment in the first 4 years of life from characteristics assessed in the neonatal period. *Child Abuse and Neglect, 23*(4), 305–319.

Kotchick, B. A., & Forehand, R. (2002). Putting parenting in perspective: A discussion of the contextual factors that shape parenting practices. *Journal of Child and Family Studies, 11*(3), 255–269.

Lee, Y. (2009). Early motherhood and harsh parenting: The role of human, social, and cultural capital. *Child Abuse and Neglect, 33*(9), 625–637.

Lee, Y., & Guterman, N. B. (2010). Young mother–father dyads and maternal harsh parenting behavior. *Child Abuse and Neglect, 34*(11), 874–885.

Lee, B. J., & Goerge, R. M. (1999). Poverty, early childbearing, and child maltreatment: A multinomial analysis. *Children and Youth Services Review, 21*(9), 755–780.

Leve, L. D., Khurana, A., & Reich, E. B. (2015). Intergenerational transmission of maltreatment: A multilevel examination. *Development and Psychopathology, 27*, 1429–1442.

Li, F., Godinet, M. T., & Arnsberger, P. (2011). Protective factors among families with children at risk of maltreatment: Follow up to early school years. *Children and Youth Services Review, 33*, 139–148.

Leventhal, J. M., Egerter, S. A., & Murphy, J. M. (1984). Reassessment of the relationship of perinatal risk factors and child abuse. *American Journal of Diseases of Children, 138*(11), 1034–1039.

Locke, T. F., & Newcomb, M. D. (2003). Childhood maltreatment, parental alcohol/drug-related problems, and global parental dysfunction. *Professional Psychology: Research and Practice, 34*, 73–79.

Lynch, M., & Cicchetti, D. Links between community violence and the family systems: Evidence from children's feelings of relatedness and perceptions of parental behavior. *Family Process, 41*(3), 519-532.

Lynch, M. A., & Roberts, J. (1977). Predicting child abuse: Signs of bonding failure in the maternity hospital. *British Medical Journal, 1*(6061), 624–626.

MacMillan, H. L., Fleming, J. E., Streiner, D. L., Lin, E., Boyle, M. H., Jamieson, E., … & Beardslee, W. R. (2001). Childhood abuse and lifetime psychopathology in a community sample. *American Journal of Psychiatry, 158*(11), 1878–1883.

Maguire-Jack, K. (2014). Multilevel investigation into the community context of child maltreatment. *Journal of Aggression, Maltreatment & Trauma, 23*(3), 229–248.

Mersky, J. P., Berger, L. M., Reynolds, A. J., & Gromoske, A. N. (2009). Risk factors for child and adolescent maltreatment: A longitudinal investigation of a cohort of inner-city youth. *Child Maltreatment, 14*(1), 73–88.

Moor, A., & Silvern, L. (2006). Identifying pathways linking child abuse to psychological outcome: The mediating role of perceived parental failure of empathy. *Journal of Emotional Abuse, 6*(4), 91–114.

Moffitt, T. E., & Caspi, A. (2003). Preventing the intergenerational continuity of antisocial behaviour: Implications of partner violence. *Early Prevention of Adult Antisocial Behaviour*, 109–129.

Neppl, T. K., Conger, R. D., Scaramella, L. V., & Ontai, L. L. (2009). Intergenerational continuity in parenting behavior: Mediating pathways and child effects. *Developmental Psychology, 45*(5), 1241.

Pears, K. C., & Capaldi, D. M. (2001). Intergenerational transmission of abuse: A two-generational prospective study of an at-risk sample. *Child Abuse and Neglect, 25*(11), 1439–1461.

Putnam, S. P., Sanson, A. V., & Rothbart, M. K. (2002). Child temperament and parenting. *Handbook of Parenting, 1*, 255–277.

Radey, M., Schelbe, L., McWey, L. M., Holtrop, K., & Canto, A. I. (2016). "It's really overwhelming": Parent and service provider perspectives of parents aging out of foster care. *Children and Youth Services Review, 67*, 1–10.

Renner, L., & Slack, K. S. (2006). Intimate partner violence and child maltreatment: Understanding intra- and intergenerational connections. *Child Abuse & Neglect,30*(6), 599–617.

Runyan, D. K., Hunter, W. M., Socolar, R. R., Amaya-Jackson, L., English, D., Landsverk, J., et al. (1998). Children who prosper in unfavorable environments: The relationship to social capital. *Pediatrics, 101*(1), 12–18.

Scaramella, L. V., & Conger, R. D. (2003). Intergenerational continuity of hostile parenting and its consequences: The moderating influence of children's negative emotional reactivity. *Social Development, 12*(3), 420–439.

Sheppard, M. (1997). Double jeopardy: The link between child abuse and maternal depression in child and family social work. *Child and Family Social Work, 2*, 91–107.

Sidebotham, P., Heron, J., & ALSPAC Study Team. (2006). Child maltreatment in the "children of the nineties": A cohort study of risk factors. *Child Abuse & Neglect, 30*(5), 497–522.

Sidebotham, P., Golding, J., & ALSPAC Study Team. (2001). Child maltreatment in the "Children of the Nineties": A longitudinal study of parental risk factors. *Child Abuse & Neglect, 25*(9), 1177–1200.

Smith, C. A., Ireland, T. O., Park, A., Elwyn, L., & Thornberry, T. P. (2011). Intergenerational continuities and discontinuities in intimate partner violence: A two-generation prospective study. *Journal of Interpersonal Violence, 26*, 3720–3752.

Smith, J. A. S., & Adler, R. G. (1991). Children hospitalized with child abuse and neglect: A case-control study. *Child Abuse and Neglect, 15*(4), 437–445.

Skuse, D. H., Gill, D., Reilly, S., Wolke, D., & Lynch, M. A. (1995). Failure to thrive and the risk of child abuse: A prospective population survey. *Journal of Medical Screening, 2*(3), 145–149.

Stevens-Simon, C., Nelligan, D., & Kelly, L. (2001). Adolescents at risk for mistreating their children: Part II: A home-and clinic-based prevention program. *Child Abuse and Neglect, 25*(6), 753–769.

Straus, M. A. (1979). Family patterns and child abuse in a nationally representative American sample. *Child Abuse and Neglect, 3*(1), 213–225.

Tempel, L. R. (2007). Pathways to the clinician's experience of empathy in engaging single mothers at risk for physical abuse of their children. *Clinical Social Work Journal, 35*(4), 257–265.

Thompson, R. (2006). Exploring the link between maternal history of childhood victimization and child risk of maltreatment. *Journal of Trauma Practice, 5*(2), 57–72.

Thornberry, T. P., & Henry, K. L. (2013). Intergenerational continuity in maltreatment. *Journal of Abnormal Child Psychology, 41*(4), 555–569.

Thornberry, T. P., Freeman-Gallant, A., Lizotte, A. J., Krohn, M. D., & Smith, C. A. (2003). Linked lives: The intergenerational transmission of antisocial behavior. *Journal of Abnormal Child Psychology, 31*(2), 171–184.

Valentino, K., Nuttall, A., Comas, M., Borkowski, J., & Akai, C. (2012). Intergenerational continuity of child abuse among adolescent mothers: Authoritarian parenting, community violence, and race. *Child Maltreatment, 17*, 172–181.

Walsh, C., MacMillan, H., & Jamieson, E. (2002). The relationship between parental psychiatric disorder and child physical and sexual abuse: Findings from the Ontario Health Supplement. *Child Abuse and Neglect, 26*(2), 11–22.

Widom, C. S., DuMont, K., & Czaja, S. J. (2007). A prospective investigation of major depressive disorder and comorbidity in abused and neglected children grown up. *Archives of General Psychiatry, 64*(1), 49–56.

Widom, C. S., Czaja, S. J., & DuMont, K. A. (2015). Intergenerational transmission of child abuse and neglect: Real or detection bias? *Science, 347*(6229), 1480–1485.

Widom, C. S., Czaja, S., & Dutton, M. A. (2014). Child abuse and neglect and intimate partner violence victimization and perpetration: A prospective investigation. *Child Abuse and Neglect, 38*(4), 650–663.

Wiehe, V. R. (1997). Approaching child abuse treatment from the perspective of empathy. *Child Abuse and Neglect, 21*(12), 1191–1204.

Whitson, M. L., Martinez, A., Ayala, C., & Kaufman, J. S. (2011). Predictors of parenting and infant outcomes for impoverished adolescent parents. *Journal of Family Social Work, 14*(4), 284–297.

Zielinski, D. S., & Bradshaw, C. P. (2006). Ecological influences on the sequelae of child maltreatment: A review of the literature. *Child Maltreatment, 11*(1), 49–62.

Chapter 5
Interrupting Intergenerational Transmission of Child Maltreatment: Protective Factors Associated with Breaking the Cycle of Maltreatment

5.1 Resilience and Protective Factors

The concept of resilience was developed following an examination of individuals and groups who were able to "overcome the odds" and do well in light of adversity (e.g., Masten et al. 1990; Werner and Smith 1992). Resilience is a dynamic process of adapting well in the face of adversity, trauma, tragedy, threats, or significant sources of stress—such as family and relationship problems, serious health problems, or other stressors (Luthar et al. 2000). It is often referred to as "bouncing back" from difficult experiences. Resilience is common and can be manifested in many ways. It does not mean that a person who is resilient does not have negative or difficult experiences, but rather the person possesses more traits and skills that help to manage stressors associated with difficult experiences.

Early resilience research focused more on individual traits. Rutter (1987) describes the interaction between one's individual traits and the environment. This line of research began to inform how relationships can serve as a contributor to individual and family resilience (Walsh 2006). Key relationships with romantic partners, parents, peers, and other supportive adults helped improve individual and family well-being. Research has identified several factors that promote resilience in individuals. For example, social support and positive relationships, insight, independence, initiative, creativity and humor, and morality or spirituality have been identified as key factors that contribute to individual and family resilience (Lietz 2006; Walsh 2006; Wolin and Wolin 1993). These factors and processes have been shown to be successful in promoting resilience and drawing on one's strengths, abilities, and resources across various groups of people experiencing adversity, such as substance abuse, child maltreatment, and family violence.

Protective factors are internal or external resources that may buffer or modify the impact of specific risk factors (Rutter 1987). Garmezy (1985) identified three broad categories of protective factors: individual attributes, family milieu, and extra-familial social environment. Individual attributes include temperament, cognitive

L. Schelbe and J.M. Geiger, *Intergenerational Transmission of Child Maltreatment*, SpringerBriefs in Social Work,
DOI 10.1007/978-3-319-43824-5_5

abilities, and coping skills. Family can influence an individual's well-being by providing safety, support, and warmth. A person's social environment contributes social supports and other resources that can enhance well-being. The two most influential protective factors that promote resilience throughout childhood are the presence of a strong prosocial relationship with at least one caring adult and having good intellectual capabilities (Rutter 1987; Werner and Smith 1982). Protective factors, as with risk factors, may exist within a specific domain and do not necessarily apply to an individual's overall well-being. Thornberry and colleagues (2013) explain that "a direct protective factor is a variable that decreases the likelihood or level of a problematic outcome among those at risk," however, "a buffering protective factor is a variable that significantly offsets the harmful effects of a risk factor (e.g., maltreatment) on an outcome (e.g., perpetration)" (p. S28).

Across a variety of disciplines and areas of research and practice fields, there is a growing interest in the concept of resilience and how we can promote, teach, and cultivate it in individuals, families, and communities. There are several ecological factors that have been shown to protect against child maltreatment and ITCM. Protective factors may diminish the negative impact of risk factors and are not simply the absence of risk factors (Garmezy 1985; Rutter 1987). For example, relationships, education, delaying pregnancy/parenting, and social support seem to moderate the cycle or continuity of child maltreatment into subsequent generations. Some of the research refers to those who have not continued the cycle of ITCM as "cycle breakers." When attempting to tease out some of the factors that have interrupted the cycle of maltreatment, several individual, familial, and community factors have been examined. Studies continue to have mixed findings, with no definitive pathway to prevent ITCM.

The following is an overview and discussion of the factors associated with positive parenting and protective factors related to the parent, involving social support and relationships, and community components that may help to reduce ITCM and child maltreatment.

5.2 Parental Resilience and Protective Factors

Individual traits such as personality, parenting skills, and the ability to "cognitively reframe" the experience of child maltreatment can help to disrupt ITCM. Parental resilience refers to the ability of parents to cope effectively with the stressors and challenges associated with parenting children. Parental resilience often includes a parent's emotional and mental health, decision-making skills, empathy, and meeting the needs of their child or children in light of adversity. Skills such as accessing resources, obtaining needed social support, and managing stress effectively also contribute to parental resilience. For parents who have experienced child maltreatment, these attributes and skills can help to buffer the effects of their experiences of child maltreatment and to help prevent ITCM. Studies have also shown that parents who have knowledge about child development and who have appropriate expectations of children can better understand and manage children's behaviors and emotions, in turn contributing to a child's well-being (Shonkoff and Phillips 2000). Parental competence and balancing appropriate discipline, warmth, empathy, and care are essential to healthy caregiving (Schaffer et al. 2009).

When parents have this knowledge and ability, they may be able to parent more effectively in spite of their experiences of parenting, which may be negative. Early research has also shown that decisions prior to parenthood (e.g., attitudes toward pregnancy, likeliness to obtain prenatal care, and increased social resources) can also have an influence on ITCM (Hunter and Kilstrom 1979). An individual's choice to delay pregnancy and parenthood (age) can also reduce the likelihood of ITCM (Bartlett and Easterbrooks 2015).

Financial security has also been associated with reducing the effects of a parent's experience of childhood maltreatment (Dixon et al. 2009). Financial problems are often the source of stress for parents and families as well as tension and discord between spouses/partners. When financial security exists within a family, stress is reduced and children are at a lower risk of maltreatment. Financial security may also be associated with an increased ability to provide for one's family's basic needs and a safer living environment, thereby reducing the risk of maltreatment and ITCM. Education may also have the potential to lead to increased financial security and has also been shown to buffer the effects of child maltreatment and ITCM.

Parents who have experienced childhood maltreatment have also been shown to be extremely resilient despite their experiences and others' expectations of them as parents and individuals. Notwithstanding statistics documenting ITCM, many parents with a history of child maltreatment do not go on to continue the cycle of maltreatment with their own children. Herrenkohl (2013) describes the study of resilience among children who have experienced violence. Individuals who have experienced maltreatment and violence often show incredible amounts of resilience in the form of emotional intelligence, empathy, initiative and motivation, and insight (Klika and Herrenkohl 2013). Such individual traits and abilities are innate and learned in light of positive and negative childhood experience. Many involve the support of other individuals and communities.

5.3 Child Resilience and Protective Factors

A child's ability to overcome the negative effects of the experience of child maltreatment also plays a role in reducing the incidence of ITCM. A child's behavior or reaction to maltreatment can also be protective. For example, adolescent aggressive behavior/externalizing behavior has been shown to act as a protective factor (Hops et al. 2003). Furthermore, a child's social and emotional competence and communication skills can act as a protective factor against child maltreatment as they often increase the strength of the child–caregiver relationship (Widom 1989). A child's behavior should never be considered a cause of maltreatment; however, it could point to family dysfunction, and negative behavior can lead to stress and unhealthy discipline practices (Walsh et al. 2015). A child's resilience and social emotional abilities can lead to early reporting and engagement in services to help with reducing mental health problems associated with the experience of child maltreatment.

5.4 Family Level Protective Factors

Social support from family, friends, and other formal and informal sources are keys in reducing child maltreatment and ITCM (e.g., Dixon et al. 2009; Egeland et al. 1988; Institute of Medicine 2014; Shaw and Kilburn 2009). Several studies cite formal and informal social support as the most effective means to reducing the incidence of child maltreatment among those parents who have experienced maltreatment themselves. Having social networks that lead to useful resources and support is also important in healthy parenting experiences.

Interpersonal processes and relationships have also been shown to be strong influences in preventing ITCM. When examining the relationship between parents or a parent and their partner, warmth and positive communication help to promote positive parenting practices, thus reducing the risk of maltreatment (e.g., Conger et al. 2013; Jaffee et al. 2013; Thornberry et al. 2013). The presence of a partner and/or a parent being married has also been shown to be a protective factor in ITCM literature (e.g., Egeland et al. 1988; Li et al. 2011). Conger and colleagues (2013) found that warm and positive communication by partners reduced the continuity of harsh parenting and nurturing behaviors of one's partner completely disrupted continuity of harsh parenting. A study by Jaffee and colleagues (2013) and Thornberry and colleagues (2013) also showed that supportive partners may facilitate the process of cycle breaking (vs. cycle maintaining) and note that there are differences with relationships among family members rather than relationships outside the family. Early research in the ITCM literature, Egeland and colleagues (1988) point to stable and satisfying relationships as a variable that buffered the effects of childhood maltreatment and ITCM.

The relationship between the parent and child also plays a role in buffering the risks associated with ITCM. For example, in a 2013 special issue of the Journal of Adolescent Health, researchers discussed ITCM and reported on studies that examined factors identified by the CDC as safe, stable, and nurturing relationships (SSNRs) and their mediating effects with a history of child maltreatment and the incidence of ITCM. The majority of the studies included in the special issue conclude that all or some of the SSNRs show an impact on reducing ITCM. For example, Herrenkohl and colleagues (2013) found that parents who had had a caring relationship with their father had reduced odds of using harsh parenting. However, Thornberry and colleagues (2013) did not find support for current attachment to and support from a person's primary caregiver during adolescence, thus concluded "not all positive relationships provide preventative benefits" (p. S29). They found that three out of the five SSNRs (relationship satisfaction, parental satisfaction, and attachment to child) served as protective factors for ITCM. Schofield and colleagues (2013) conducted a meta-analysis of SSNRs as a moderator of intergenerational continuity of child maltreatment and found that SSNRs do, in fact, disrupt the intergenerational cycle of maltreatment. SSNRs included in the five studies evaluated were emotional intimacy, trust, social support, partner warmth and support, communication, relationship satisfaction, parenting satisfaction, and parental attachment and support (Schofield et al. 2013).

In the early 2000s, the Center for the Study of Social Policy (CSSP) created a framework for building strengths within families and that also promotes a partnership between families and organizations that focuses more on individual and family strengths versus identified risks (Horton 2011). Similar to the CDC's SSNRs, CSSP identified five evidence-based protective factors that have been shown to reduce child maltreatment; namely, parental resilience, social connections, knowledge of parenting and child development, concrete support, and social and emotional competence of children. The U.S. Administration on Children, Youth, and Families (ACYF) also adopted an approach based on this framework that highlighted several factors that have been shown to protect children from the effects of maltreatment. These protective factors related to the individual, relationships, and the community, include: self-regulation, parenting competence, positive relationships, and stable environment (Horton 2011).

Child maltreatment continues to be a serious public health concern. Examining and implementing ways to promote healthy children and families through SSNRs, communities, and programs is a key to beginning to prevent and address child maltreatment and its deleterious effects. These relationships and protective factors can also be effective in addressing ITCM (Conger et al. 2013; Herrenkohl et al. 2013; Schofield et al. 2013; Thornberry et al. 2013). The Centers for Disease Control and Prevention (CDC) are committed to examining and promoting SSNRs between children and their caregivers through funding, research, and programmatic support (CDC 2014). The CDC established three dimensions of relationships (safety, stability, nurturing) that are critical in the child and family's environment to promote well-being and healthy development. In their efforts to promote SSNRs to prevent child maltreatment and ITCM, the CDC focuses on: educating parents and caregivers, providing concrete and emotional social support, and embedding a framework for agencies and organizations serving children and families who may be at a greater risk for maltreatment.

5.5 Community Protective Factors

Community, programs, and other social supports are also believed to buffer the potential for negative outcomes associated with child maltreatment and ITCM. Several federal and state agencies have adopted programs to address child maltreatment and ITCM by providing economic and concrete support programs and policies (Daro and Dodge 2009). Community resilience is a newer concept to encourage members to work together to support families and children in an effort to reduce child maltreatment. Other community level strategies include: early intervention programs for children and families, more community program and school engagement with parents and families, and facilitating relationships and dialogue among parents and caregivers to foster support and access to resources and programs.

The CDC developed a guide for promoting local and state efforts to ensure SSNRs on a community level (CDC 2014). The framework includes four overarching goals: (1) raising awareness and commitment to promoting SSNRs in communities, (2) using research and data to inform programming, (3) using policy and legislation to promote child and family well-being, and (4) creating a context for healthy children and families by changing norms and expectations. The *Essentials for Childhood* framework aims to use a widespread, far-reaching inclusive approach to reducing child maltreatment, and in turn ITCM (CDC 2014).

5.6 Caution and Considerations

While protective factors are important to consider while trying to understand ITCM, it cannot be assumed that all protective factors are the same for different groups of people. For example, Valentino and colleagues (2012) found authoritarian parenting attitudes for African American mothers was a protective factor for their children's maltreatment, although the same was not true for Caucasian mothers. The authors explain that one of the reasons for African American mothers holding authoritarian parenting attitudes is protective in that the daily threats in their environment are real and that controlling children is both adaptive and appropriate. This example can remind us of the importance of taking context and culture into consideration when examining protective factors and not making the assumption that protective factors will be the same for all people. As so much remains unknown in the etiology and in ITCM, caution should be exercised in drawing conclusions about how protective factors interact and for which populations the protective factors are relevant.

5.7 Conclusion

Not all parents who experience maltreatment go onto abuse their children. There is a constellation of protective factors that may contribute to this. Research has found various factors at different levels (e.g., individual, family, and community) contribute to interrupting the cycle of violence. As we discuss in Chap. 7, intervention and prevention strategies can incorporate the knowledge about protective factors into programs designed to prevent child maltreatment and ITCM. Future research is needed to understand protective factors, differences among groups, and interactions among protective factors.

References

Bartlett, J. D., & Easterbrooks, M. A. (2015). The moderating effect of relationships on intergenerational risk for infant neglect by young mothers. *Child Abuse and Neglect, 45*, 21–34.

Center for Study of Social Policy. (2016). Strengthening families: The protective factors framework. Retrieved from: http://www.cssp.org/reform/strengthening-families/basic-one-pagers/Strengthening-Families-Protective-Factors.pdf

Centers for Disease Control and Prevention. (2014). Essentials for childhood framework: Steps to create safe, stable, nurturing relationships and environments for all children. Retrieved from: http://www.cdc.gov/violenceprevention/childmaltreatment/essentials.html

Conger, R. D., Schofield, T. J., Neppl, T. K., & Merrick, M. T. (2013). Disrupting intergenerational continuity in harsh and abusive parenting: The importance of a nurturing relationship with a romantic partner. *Journal of Adolescent Health, 53*(4), S11–S17.

Daro, D., & Dodge, K. A. (2009). Creating community responsibility for child protection: Possibilities and challenges. *Future of Children, 19*(2), 67–93.

Dixon, L., Browne, K., & Hamilton-Giachritsis, C. (2009). Patterns of risk and protective factors in the intergenerational cycle of maltreatment. *Journal of Family Violence, 24*(2), 111–122.

Egeland, B., Jacobvitz, D., & Sroufe, L. A. (1988). Breaking the cycle of abuse. *Child Development*, 1080–1088.

Garmezy, N. (1985). Stress-resistant children: The search for protective factors. *Recent Research in Developmental Psychopathology, 4*, 213–233.

Herrenkohl, T. I. (2013). Person–environment interactions and the shaping of resilience. *Trauma, Violence, & Abuse, 14*(3), 191–194.

Herrenkohl, T. I., Klika, J. B., Brown, E. C., Herrenkohl, R. C., & Leeb, R. T. (2013). Tests of the mitigating effects of caring and supportive relationships in the study of abusive disciplining over two generations. *Journal of Adolescent Health, 53*(4), S18–S24.

Hops, H., Davis, B., Leve, C., & Sheeber, L. (2003). Cross-generational transmission of aggressive parent behavior: A prospective, mediational examination. *Journal of Abnormal Child Psychology, 31*(2), 161–169.

Horton, C. (2011). Protective factors literature review: Early care and education programs and the prevention of child abuse and neglect. Retrieved from: http://www.cssp.org/reform/strengthening-families/resources/body/LiteratureReview.pdf

Hunter, R. S., & Kilstrom, N. (1979). Breaking the cycle in abusive families. *The American Journal of Psychiatry, 136*(10), 1320–1322.

Institute of Medicine and National Research Council. (2014). *New directions in child abuse and neglect research*. Washington, DC: The National Academies Press.

Jaffee, S. R., Bowes, L., Ouellet-Morin, I., Fisher, H. L., Moffitt, T. E., Merrick, M. T., & Arseneault, L. (2013). Safe, stable, nurturing relationships break the intergenerational cycle of abuse: A prospective nationally representative cohort of children in the United Kingdom. *Journal of Adolescent Health, 53*(4), S4–S10.

Klika, J. B., & Herrenkohl, T. I. (2013). A review of developmental research on resilience in maltreated children. *Trauma, Violence, & Abuse, 14*(3), 222–234.

Li, F., Godinet, M. T., & Arnsberger, P. (2011). Protective factors among families with children at risk of maltreatment: Follow up to early school years. *Children and Youth Services Review, 33*, 139–148.

Lietz, C. (2006). Uncovering stories of family resilience: A mixed methods study of resilient families, part 1. *Families in Society: The Journal of Contemporary Social Services, 87*(4), 575–582.

Luthar, S. S., Cicchetti, D., & Becker, B. (2000). The construct of resilience: A critical evaluation and guidelines for future work. *Child Development, 71*(3), 543–562.

Masten, A. S., Best, K. M., & Garmezy, N. (1990). Resilience and development: Contributions from the study of children who overcome adversity. *Development and Psychopathology, 2*(04), 425–444.

Rutter, M. (1987). Psychosocial resilience and protective mechanisms. *American Journal of Orthopsychiatry, 57*(3), 316.

Schaffer, M., Clark, S., & Jeglic, E. L. (2009). The role of empathy and parenting style in the development of antisocial behaviors. *Crime & Delinquency, 55*(4), 586–599.

Schofield, T. J., Lee, R. D., & Merrick, M. T. (2013). Safe, stable, nurturing relationships as a moderator of intergenerational continuity of child maltreatment: A meta-analysis. *Journal of Adolescent Health, 53*(4), S32–S38.

Shaw, R., & Kilburn, M. (2009). Child abuse and neglect prevention: Reports from the Field and Ideas for the Future. Unpublished document prepared for the Doris Duke Foundation. Retrieved August 5, 2011, from. http://www.rand.org/pubs/working_papers/2009/RAND_WR632.pdf

Shonkoff, J. P., & Phillips, D. A. (Eds.). (2000). *From neurons to neighborhoods: The science of early childhood development.* Washington, D.C.: National Academies Press.

Thornberry, T. P., Henry, K. L., Smith, C. A., Ireland, T. O., Greenman, S. J., & Lee, R. D. (2013). Breaking the cycle of maltreatment: The role of safe, stable, and nurturing relationships. *Journal of Adolescent Health, 53*(4), S25–S31.

Valentino, K., Nuttall, A., Comas, M., Borkowski, J., & Akai, C. (2012). Intergenerational continuity of child abuse among adolescent mothers: Authoritarian parenting, community violence, and race. *Child Maltreatment, 17*, 172–181.

Walsh, F. (2006). *Strengthening family resilience* (2nd ed.). New York: Guilford Press.

Walsh, T. B., McCourt, S. N., Rostad, W. L., Byers, K., & Ocasio, K. (2015). Promoting protective factors and strengthening resilience. In D. Daro, A. C. Donnelly, L. A. Huang, & B. J. Powell (Eds.), *Advances in child abuse prevention knowledge* (pp. 203–233). New York: Springer International Publishing.

Werner, E. E., & Smith, R. S. (1982). Vulnerable but not invincible: A study of resilient children.

Werner, E. E., & Smith, R. S. (1992). *Overcoming the odds: High risk children from birth to adulthood.* USA: Cornell University Press.

Widom, C. S. (1989). Child abuse, neglect, and adult behavior: Research design and findings on criminality, violence, and child abuse. *American Journal of Orthopsychiatry, 59*(3), 355–367.

Wolin, S., & Wolin, S. (1993). The resilient self: How survivors of troubled families rise above adversity. New York: Villard.

Chapter 6
Future Research on Intergenerational Transmission of Child Maltreatment: Methods, Constructs, and Contexts

6.1 Intergenerational Transmission of Child Maltreatment Research

Child maltreatment and the intergenerational transmission of child maltreatment (ITCM) have been studied for many decades, yet we still do not fully understand the causes and mechanisms through which parents maltreat their children. We do not know why some parents who were maltreated as children continue the cycle of violence in their family while others are able to break the cycle and discontinue ITCM. The research is extensive, but we only have the most basic understanding of the phenomenon. In Chap. 3, we reviewed the research on ITCM and highlighted the limitations of previous research. This chapter expands upon the limitations discussed and offers specific guidance for future research questions as well as designs and methods that will help understand the complexity of ITCM.

Scholars who investigate ITCM offer various recommendations about what should be done in future research about ITCM. As several have noted, the great proportion of ITCM literature has been review articles rather than empirical pieces (Ertem et al. 2000; Thornberry et al. 2012). These review articles included specific guidelines for future research. Ertem and colleagues (2000) as well as Thornberry and colleagues (2012) in their systematic reviews outlined methodological standards by which to assess ITCM research as well as to guide future research. (See Table 6.1 which compares the standards proposed by the systematic reviews. This table summarizes the methodological standards that systematic reviews of ITCM studies have used to evaluate empirical studies.) These guidelines, as well as the recommendations from empirical articles, can assist with creating an agenda for future ITCM research.

L. Schelbe and J.M. Geiger, *Intergenerational Transmission of Child Maltreatment*, SpringerBriefs in Social Work,
DOI 10.1007/978-3-319-43824-5_6

Table 6.1 Methodological standards for evaluating intergenerational transmission of child maltreatment in review studies

Category of standards	Ertem et al. (2000)	Thornberry et al. (2012)
Clear definition of maltreatment	Clear description of abuse	A clear definition of maltreatment
Measurement of maltreatment	Clear description of person who abused G2 Clear definition of outcome	Measure of maltreatment with proven validity and reliability Different reporters of maltreatment for each generation
Considering other factors	Adequate control for intervening variable	Controls for antecedent factors that may cause spurious relationships
Sampling	Equal demographic and clinical susceptibility	A sample that is representative of a general population Maltreated and non-maltreated sample members in the focal generation A satisfactory participation rate and low levels of attrition
Control/comparison group	Ensuring nonabuse of controls	Assessment of maltreatment status for the comparison group
Data sources	Avoidance of recall and detection bias	Prospective data
Research design	Equal surveillance of both groups for the outcome event	The same exposure period for treatment and comparison Follow-up over an extended portion of the life course

6.2 Areas of Inquiry

Kaufman and Zigler (1987) concluded their review of ITCM literature calling for research to move beyond simple confirmation of the cycle of violence hypotheses: "The time has come for the intergenerational myth to be placed aside; and for researchers to cease to ask, 'Do abused children become abusive parents?' Instead, they urge researchers to ask, 'Under what conditions is the transmission of abuse most likely to occur?'" (p. 191). While this call for action in research is now almost 30-years old, it remains relevant today. At that time and up until now, studies continue to be published showing the occurrence of ITCM, while few are examining the mechanisms and context for ITCM.

6.2.1 Mechanisms

Very limited knowledge exists about the specific mechanisms that can disrupt ITCM (Conger et al. 2013). Nor is there adequate knowledge about the mechanisms through which ITCM continues. As such, future research should examine both

(Berzenski et al. 2014). Herzberger (1990) stresses the need for future research to ask, "What forms of maltreatment lead to maltreatment of others, and can one form of maltreatment lead to another form?" (p. 537).

We need to identify models that can explain ITCM (Dixon et al. 2005a; Neugebauer 2000). This can ultimately help develop appropriate interventions to be created to break the cycle (Dixon et al. 2005a). Examining those who break the cycle and those who discontinue ITCM is important (Herzberger 1990), both within the context of interventions and independently. As there is some evidence of homotypic ITCM, studies should look at mechanisms that are specific to types of maltreatment (Berzenski et al. 2014). Currently, there is insufficient research to determine homotypic or heterotypic transmission patterns. As we will discuss below, understanding specific types of maltreatment and ITCM is important and may be crucial to understanding the mechanisms of ITCM (Berzenski et al. 2014).

6.2.2 *Theory*

Theory can guide research and can contribute to framing studies and interpreting results. There is a need to integrate and develop theory within ITCM research (Geiger et al. 2015). As discussed in Chap. 2, there are multiple theories that can be useful to understanding ITCM. Theory can identify factors that contribute to ITCM (Dixon et al. 2005a). Widom and Wilson (2015) argue "Future research needs to adopt ecological models that consider the individual in the context of the broader social environment in which he or she functions" (p. 41). Studies should examine individual levels such as development and levels of functioning (Berzenski et al. 2014), family levels, as well as neighborhood and macro levels.

6.2.3 *Program Evaluation*

As we will discuss in Chap. 7, prevention and intervention strategies can address ITCM and attempt to break the cycle of violence. These efforts should be evaluated so that we can determine what works for whom in what context. Ensuring that culture, race, and ethnicity are addressed in all areas of child maltreatment research is critical (Institute of Medicine and National Research Council 2014). Understanding which programs can potentially discontinue maltreatment can help inform resource allocation to make the largest impact.

6.3 Methods

Clearly a randomized control trial cannot be conducted with children randomly assigned to a maltreatment or control group (Widom and Wilson 2015). Whereas the "gold standard" of a randomized control trial is not an option for research, other methods can further our knowledge about ITCM and child maltreatment in general. Research methods must go beyond providing simple descriptive data and rates of transmission. Multivariate and multilevel analyses are needed (Herzberger 1990; Leve et al. 2015) as are more correlational studies required to test causal models (Widom 2015).

Future research should use longitudinal studies (Neugebauer 2000), specifically prospective cohort studies. Participants should be enrolled prior to the birth of a child (Widom 2015) and followed for generations. Studies should use probability samples drawn from a well-defined population (Thornberry et al. 2012) and ideally, be nationally representative.

Qualitative studies can contribute to the knowledge about ITCM. Understanding differences between "cycle breakers" and "cycle maintainers" can have important ramifications for understanding the processes and mechanisms of ITCM. It is likely that there is not a single pathway from being maltreated as a child and continuation of maltreatment within future generations nor a single pathway of breaking the cycle, and understanding possible typologies and patterns can be best explored through qualitative methods (McWey et al. 2013). Obtaining the perspectives and input from those who have experienced childhood maltreatment and who have continued and discontinued ITCM can be extremely valuable in better understanding the processes and mechanisms of ITCM.

ITCM cannot be seen simply as a phenomenon that can be examined exclusively from a behavioral or social science lens. Future research should aim to incorporate genetics, as research that examined violent and antisocial behavior has done with different genotypes (e.g., Beaver et al. 2010; Caspi et al. 2002; Widom and Brzustowicz 2006) or interactions among genes (e.g., Beaver et al. 2007; Guo et al. 2007), or gene-environment interactions (e.g., Beaver et al. 2009; Moffitt 2005). Epigenetics and examining gene expression may also be relevant in ITCM research (Conger et al. 2009; Geiger et al. 2015). Animal analogue studies may also provide important insights about ITCM and maltreatment (Widom 2015).

6.4 Variables

More nuanced operationalization of maltreatment is needed within ITCM research. Maltreatment cannot be measured simply as a dichotomous variable. Specific aspects of maltreatment such as chronicity and severity may be important to examine (Berzenski et al. 2014). Herzberger (1990) concludes "The trick is to determine under what conditions a particular type, severity, and frequency of treatment will affect our interactions with others and in what ways" (p. 537). Further, Etter and Rickert (2013) conclude that research should include "…greater consistency in terminology, methodology, and measures used" (p. S40). There is a need to consider abuse types. For example, "…Are certain types of maltreatment worse than others with respect to long-term consequences and intergenerational continuity?" (Etter and Rickert 2013, p. S40).

Future research must examine specific types of maltreatment in ITCM research, as previous research has often either not clearly defined the types of maltreatment or has focused specifically on physical maltreatment. Specifically, more attention must be paid to neglect (Berlin et al. 2011; Berzenski et al. 2014; Lounds et al. 2006; Neugebauer 2000) and emotional abuse (Berzenski et al. 2014). Research on sexual abuse is also warranted considering that parents who experienced sexual abuse as children may not go onto sexually abuse their children, yet their children may experience other forms of maltreatment. For example, Dilillo and colleagues (2000) found that women who experienced child sexual abuse were more likely to physically abuse their children.

In considering the different types of maltreatment, there is a need to look at mechanisms specific to subtypes as mentioned above in the call to explore homotypic and heterotypic ITCM. However, it is important to remember that there is high comorbidity in types of maltreatment, thus it may be challenging to examine the specificity and to explore differences among different types of maltreatment (Berzenski et al. 2014). Likewise, there are studies that have found links between parents experiencing one type of maltreatment and their children experiencing another as is the case with Dilillo and colleagues (2000) examination of parents' experience of child sexual abuse and the physical abuse of their children.

It is problematic to only consider substantiated cases of maltreatment as this excludes cases that were unreported or not substantiated but could still include elements of abuse and neglect. ITCM research can be strengthened through using multiple data sources to measure maltreatment (Thornberry et al. 2012). For example, studies can use officially reported cases of child maltreatment as well as self-reports (Neugebauer 2000). Future research should minimize the use of retrospective designs—especially those with long recall times (Thornberry et al. 2012).

It is also important to take into consideration other factors related to maltreatment. Which parent or caregiver was the perpetrator? Was child maltreatment when the parent was a child reported to child protective services? What were the parent's experiences in the child welfare system? As a child, was the parent removed from the home and placed in out of home care? How long was did the parent spend in out of home placement as a child? How many placements (how much placement instability) did the parent experience as a child? As a child, was the parent reunified with family? Did the parent age out of the child welfare system? It is important to understand intervening factors children faced and how they impact ITCM (Etter and Rickert 2013).

Studies need to control for potentially confounding variables (Thornberry et al. 2012). It is important to take into consideration other explanations and variables that can explain the outcomes. For example, studies should take into consideration other risk factors documented as risk and protective factors at the individual, family, and societal level. (See Chaps. 4 and 5 for information about risk and protective factors.) Specifically, Neugebauer (2000) suggests researchers "control for other childhood adversities, psychopathological behavior in the parents, and socioeconomic, non-familial environment, ecological and biological (including prenatal) factors" (p. 1117).

Differences among people must be taken into consideration, and studies should control for individual characteristics such as parents' sex and race/ethnicity (Widom 2015). It is important to examine how women and men's experiences and potential mechanisms for continuity, as well as discontinuity, are different. Many studies have explicitly examined ITCM with mothers (e.g., Berlin et al. 2011; Cort et al. 2011; Thompson 2006; Valentino et al. 2012), and other studies have controlled for and examined potential gender differences (e.g., Herrenkohl et al. 2013; Heyman and Smith Slep 2002; Hunter and Kilstrom 1979; Newcomb and Locke 2001; Sidebotham et al. 2001). Ball (2009) conducted one of the few studies specifically examining ITCM with men. More research is needed to examine gender in depth.

It is also important to explore the extent and mechanisms of ITCM in populations of people from different racial and ethnic backgrounds. More studies are need to focus on specific racial and ethnic groups such as the studies with African American samples (e.g., Leifer et al. 2004; Valentino et al. 2012) and Frias-Armenta's (2002) examination of Mexican women. ITCM research should take culture and cultural context into consideration (Baumrind 1994; Kim 2012; Widom 2015). (See Institute of Medicine and National Research Council (2014) for extended discussion about race, ethnicity, and culture in child maltreatment research.) Caution must be taken to ensure that conclusions do not perpetuate negative or prejudice stereotypes.

6.4.1 Mediators and Moderators

A mediator variable is a variable that explains a relationship between other variables, and a moderator variable is a variable that impacts the relationship strength between other variables. Within child maltreatment research, there has been more work using mediators than moderators of outcomes of child maltreatment (Herrenkohl et al. 2013). When examining ITCM, studies should take into consideration both mediators and moderators. We need to focus on variables that moderate the relationship of ITCM (Conger et al. 2009; Neugebauer 2000). Berlin and colleagues (2011), who examined three mediators (mothers' mental health problems, mothers' social isolation, and mothers' social information processing patterns) in their examination of ITCM, stress the need to explore how mediators interact with one another within ITCM research. Thornberry and colleagues (2012) conclude in their systematic review, "We first need to understand the nature and strength of the relationship between history of maltreatment and the likelihood of maltreatment perpetration. If indeed there is clear and compelling evidence of intergenerational continuity, we then need to understand the mediating processes" (p. 146). The authors also stress the need to look at moderating influence that causes discontinuity.

Risk and protective factors can be conceptualized as examples of mediators and moderators. Understanding these factors plays an important role in understanding ITCM. (See Chaps. 4 and 5, respectively, for more information on risk and protective factors.) There needs to be more clarification and deeper understanding of risk factors

(Neugebauer 2000). Research should consider factors at each ecological level (Dixon et al. 2005b). Knowing factors that contribute to ITCM and breaking the cycle at the individual, family, and community level is important. Dixon and colleagues (2009) concluded "to provide a complete explanation of the intergenerational cycle of maltreatment, research needs to explore the complex pattern of risk and protective factors" (p. 112). The work of Dixon and colleagues (2005a) examining ITCM risk factors identified parenting under the age of 21, a history of mental illness or depression, and residing with a violent adult, and a mediation analysis found these factors explaining more than half (53 %) of the total effect. Thus, there are other factors that contribute to ITCM. Future studies need to examine additional risk and protective factors as well as the interactions among the factors.

6.5 Context

Child maltreatment occurs within the family which is influenced by outside factors. We cannot examine ITCM in isolation; context must be considered. It is necessary to examine moderators outside of the parent–child dyad and to examine community and society factors (Schofield et al. 2013). Neighborhood or community factors, as well as macro-level factors, should be considered. As explained in depth in Chap. 2, using an ecological framework helps to examine "the big picture" more completely. Perhaps the most important contexts to prioritize are those which have been clearly and consistently identified as risk factors for child maltreatment.

6.5.1 Poverty

While there is insufficient evidence to conclude that poverty causes child maltreatment, it is a recognized risk factor (Institute of Medicine and National Research Council 2014). Children living in poverty are more likely to experience child maltreatment (Berger 2004; Drake and Pandey 1996; Slack et al. 2004). Neighborhood poverty has been found to be associated with higher levels of child maltreatment (Coulton et al. 2007; Merritt 2009). The quality of parenting can be negatively influenced by variables associated with poverty including life stress, socioeconomic disadvantage, parents' age at birth of child, and neighborhood quality (Conger et al. 2009). Research has found higher levels of child welfare system involvement within low socioeconomic status communities (Jonson-Reid et al. 2009). While there is likely a surveillance bias, real differences in rates of child maltreatment likely exist. Few ITCM studies have integrated the risk factor of poverty into their models; an early study by Straus (1979) focused on poverty and found lower socioeconomic status contributing to child maltreatment. Additionally, some recent studies have controlled for socioeconomic status (Ben-David et al.

2015; Conger et al. 2013; Thornberry et al. 2013). Poverty should be acknowledged as a risk factor and should be integrated into ITCM research.

6.5.2 Intimate Partner Violence

The connections between child maltreatment and intimate partner violence are well documented (Appel and Holden 1998; Smith et al. 2011). Research has examined the co-occurrence of intimate partner violence and child maltreatment as well as experiencing child maltreatment and subsequently becoming a victim or perpetrator of intimate partner violence (Appel and Holden 1998; Dong et al. 2003; Moffitt and Caspi 2003; Renner and Slack 2006; Widom et al. 2014). More information on the risk factor of intimate partner violence is provided in Chap. 4.

Intimate partner violence is an important context to consider in ITCM (Geiger et al. 2015; Renner and Slack 2006). It is important to better understand the relationships between intimate partner violence and child maltreatment. Renner and Slack (2006) recommend that future studies examine the mediating role of intimate partner violence since various forms of childhood maltreatment, including witnessing intimate partner violence, were found to be associated with intimate partner violence in adulthood as well as ITCM. Intimate partner violence should be taken into consideration as it may be a confounding variable when examining ITCM. As there are gender differences in experiencing intimate partner violence, gender should also be taken into consideration when examining intimate partner violence and ITCM.

6.5.3 Trauma

The relevance and importance of trauma in child maltreatment research is readily recognized (Institute of Medicine and National Research Council 2014). Studies have found children who experience maltreatment are at risk for living in a stressful environment and being exposed to other potentially traumatic events, including witnessing intimate partner violence, caregiver mental illness, caregiver substance abuse, and parental absence from the home (Dong et al. 2004; Felitti et al. 1998). Considering this, it is likely that parents who experienced child maltreatment have experienced other traumas.

Parents who experience trauma may be less responsive to the needs of their children (Belsky et al. 2009). Studies of women who have experienced child sexual abuse found that survivors may experience difficulties with parenting (DiLillo and Damashek 2003) and the severity of the sexual abuse may have impacted the mothers' parenting including attachment, limit setting, communication, and involvement (Seltmann and Wright 2013). Considering the impact of traumas including child maltreatment, parents who have experienced trauma may be at risk for maltreating their children. Trauma also is important in the examination of ITCM specifically (Geiger et al. 2015). Like intimate partner violence, trauma may function as a mediator and can possibly be a confounding variable when examining ITCM (Banyard et al. 2003). Also, like intimate partner violence, gender should be taken into consideration as there is some evidence that women and men experience trauma differently (Ogden et al. 2006).

6.5.4 *Mental Health and Substance Abuse*

Mental health issues and substance abuse contribute to an increased risk of child maltreatment (see Chap. 4 for more detailed information). Research has found that children who are maltreated are more likely than those who are not maltreated to have mental health issues as adults (Edwards et al. 2003; Fergusson et al. 2008; Gilbert et al. 2009; Widom 1998). Likewise, parent's mental health, specifically depression and serious mental illness, has been identified as a risk factor for child maltreatment (Brown et al. 1998; Kotch et al. 1999; Pears and Capaldi 2001). Considering these issues together, along with the limited research that has examined parental maltreatment history and parental mental health (Banyard et al. 2003; Dixon et al. 2005a, 2005b; Pears and Capaldi 2001), there is a compelling argument to focus on ensuring ITCM research includes parents' mental health in models.

Like mental health issues, research has found that children who experience maltreatment are more likely to have problems later in life with substance use (Gilbert et al. 2009; Herrenkohl et al. 2013; Jonson-Reid et al.2012; Kunitz et al. 1998). Substance abuse has been associated with child maltreatment (Brown and Anderson 1991; Chaffin et al. 1996; Locke and Newcomb 2003). Studies examining ITCM have found substance abuse problems as a factor that increases the risk of child maltreatment among parents who have experienced maltreatment themselves (Appleyard et al. 2011; Dixon et al. 2009; Jaffee et al. 2013; Kotch et al. 1999). Substance use should be included as a contextual factor in examining ITCM.

6.5.5 *Youth Aging Out*

Youth aging out of the child welfare system who are parenting may be at risk for continuing the cycle of violence (Geiger and Schelbe 2014; Radey et al. 2016). Youth aging out are a group that should be focused upon when considering ITCM (Geiger et al. 2015) as youth aging out who are parents may not only be at risk because they experienced child maltreatment, but because there may be other factors that put them at risk for perpetuating child maltreatment (e.g., adolescent parenting, poverty, low educational attainment). Thus, more research needs to focus on this specific population and the context in which youth aging out are parenting.

6.6 Methodological Challenges in Studying Intergenerational Transmission of Child Maltreatment

Methodological problems plague research on ITCM. Various scholars have outlined lists detailing the problems (e.g., Herzberger 1990; Neugebauer 2000; Newcomb and Locke 2001; Pears and Capaldi 2001; Widom 1989). This section will outline the key areas of ITCM research which have been critiqued including definitions of child abuse, sampling, research designs, comparison group use, and approach. We discuss future research and introduce the standards proposed by scholars who have systematically evaluated ITCM research (Ertem et al. 2000; Thornberry et al. 2012).

6.6.1 Defining and Measuring Child Maltreatment

One of the most significant methodological limitations of ITCM research includes inconsistent and ambiguous definitions of abuse and neglect (Widom and Wilson 2015). Varying definitions of abuse are used in ITCM studies (Pears and Capaldi 2001). Scholars have long critiqued studies which do not distinguish between maltreatment types, such as neglect and abuse, and include them in one group (Herzberger 1990; Newcomb and Locke 2001; Widom 1989). Studies often do not take into consideration the degree of victimization. Nor do they examine the frequency and severity of the maltreatment (Herzberger 1990). Thornberry and Henry (2013) posited that in addition to the timing, the type, the chronicity, and the severity of the maltreatment offered a possible explanation for the finding about the transmission of maltreatment. It is problematic to examine maltreatment as a dichotomy rather than examine it on a continuum within multiple contexts (Newcomb and Locke 2001).

One concern about the measurement of child maltreatment is that self-report and non-substantiated cases in child protective services are used (Widom 1989). There is concern that when a definition of maltreatment requires the substantiation of a case by child protective services that the standard for maltreatment is too high and may overlook some maltreatment (Newcomb and Locke 2001).

However, others have argued that measuring child maltreatment through retroactive self-report, rather than official records, is problematic due to recall bias and misrepresentation (Neugebauer 2000; Herzberger 1990; Pears and Capaldi 2001; Widom 1989). The accuracy of retrospective data is often questionable, especially when the time between inquiry and the events is great. Asking parents to recall how their parents treated them is limited, especially considering there may be a bias to justify maltreatment as a normal part of child rearing. Additionally, as a large proportion of child maltreatment occurs before the age of five, some parents may not remember maltreatment they experienced.

6.6.2 Sampling

A critique of ITCM research has been that studies use weak sampling techniques, involving convenience or opportunity samples (Widom 1989). As mentioned with the definition of child maltreatment, one main concern around sampling lies with the use of child protective service cases that are substantiated and that overlook other maltreatment (Newcomb and Locke 2001). Using samples of substantiated cases of child maltreatment may not be directly applicable to the general population as cases coming to the attention of institutions are atypical as most victimization goes unreported (Neugebauer 2000). Neugebauer (2000) further asserts that the consequences of an allegation being substantiated and going into care may contribute to an increased risk of antisocial behavior in the future. Thus, it is concerning to assume that findings which use substantiation as the only measurement of child maltreatment can be applied to people who were never involved in the child protective services.

6.6.3 Research Design

Research designs of ITCM have been heavily criticized. Clearly, the "gold standard" of research, the randomized control trial, cannot be used as it is not possible to randomly assign children to a maltreatment or a control group (Widom and Wilson 2015). Studies examining ITCM often lack control or comparison groups of non-maltreated children (Herzberger 1990; Widom 1989; Widom and Wilson 2015). Given the failure to have such groups, it is not possible to determine the base rates of child maltreatment. Neugebauer (2000) raises concerns that "sociodemographic, economic, cultural, and environmental conditions and factors that in themselves may predispose children to aggressive behavior in adulthood" (p. 1116) are correlated with parental maltreatment. Therefore, having appropriate comparison groups can determine to what extent parental history of maltreatment contributed to a subsequent generation of maltreatment.

Specifically, the cross-sectional design has been criticized (Herzberger 1990; Widom and Wilson 2015). This is largely because with cross-sectional data, retrospective accounts of parents' experience of child maltreatment are used, which can be problematic (Herzberger 1990; Pears and Capaldi 2001). Early critiques of ITCM literature were that it was largely descriptive and relied on correlational studies (Herzberger 1990; Widom 1989). Current research has moved beyond correlations, yet studies do not always incorporate the complexity of child maltreatment into the models.

Pears and Capaldi (2001) critiqued the methods in ITCM literature for failing to consider third variable explanations. Studies do not regularly examine what other factors may explain the variance. With the ex post factor nature of many of the studies, they hold little predictive power (Widom 1989). It is important to fully understand the mechanisms and processes through which a parent's history of maltreatment influences either the continuity or discontinuity of ITCM. This can then be translated to developing child maltreatment prevention and intervention strategies.

6.7 Overall Research Challenges

Conducting research examining ITCM is challenging, and Widom (2015), who has conducted research in the area for over 30 years, observed "…the challenges are enormous, and I believe, have increased over time" (p. 83). Some of the challenges with ITCM research that scholars have noted are consistent with research in general, such as challenges recruiting samples, operationalizing definitions, measurement, and establishing causality.

There are some challenges that are unique to research examining child maltreatment (MacMillan et al. 2007) that are also germane to ITCM research. Specifically, the ethical and legal issues of reporting maltreatment can raise questions and be difficult to negotiate (Widom 2015). Institutional review boards at institutions have become more legalistic about child maltreatment research, and thus it is harder to get approval for studies examining maltreatment (Institute of Medicine and National Research Council 2014; Widom 2015). There may be concerns around issues of informed consent for children as well potential harm of asking about experiences of maltreatment (MacMillan et al. 2007). As mandatory reporting creates such a formidable obstacle, researchers not focusing specifically on child maltreatment may be deterred from incorporating questions about abuse and neglect in their research (Widom 2015).

6.8 Conclusion

With the great cost of maltreatment—to children, families, communities, and society—understanding the etiology of child maltreatment and ITCM remains of utmost importance. Future research needs to ask new questions that seek answers for how, for whom, and under what conditions ITCM occurs. Questions must examine differences among unique populations and certain circumstances and contexts. Future research must better measure maltreatment in nuanced ways that take into consideration type, severity, and chronicity. Studies are increasingly employing different methods that allow research to extend beyond simple descriptive analyses. This needs to continue, despite the reality of the challenges of conducting research on child maltreatment and ITCM. It is true that parental history of maltreatment is only one of the risk factors of child maltreatment. However, in order to prevent child maltreatment, we must remain committed to understanding ITCM.

References

Appel, A. E., & Holden, G. W. (1998). The co-occurrence of spouse and physical child abuse: A review and appraisal. *Journal of Family Psychology, 12*(4), 578.

Appleyard, K., Berlin, L. J., Rosanbalm, K. D., & Dodge, K. A. (2011). Preventing early child maltreatment: Implications from a longitudinal study of maternal abuse history, substance use problems, and offspring victimization. *Prevention Science, 12*, 139e49.

Ball, J. D. (2009). Intergenerational transmission of abuse of incarcerated fathers a study of the measurement of abuse. *Journal of Family Issues, 30*(3), 371–390.

Banyard, V. L., Williams, L. M., & Siegel, J. A. (2003). The impact of complex trauma and depression on parenting: An exploration of mediating risk and protective factors. *Child Maltreatment, 8*(4), 334–349.

Baumrind, D. (1994). The social context of child maltreatment. *Family Relations*, 360–368.

Beaver, K. M., DeLisi, M., Vaughn, M. G., & Barnes, J. C. (2010). Monoamine oxidase: A genotype is associated with gang membership and weapon use. *Comprehensive Psychiatry, 51*(2), 130–134.

Beaver, K. M., DeLisi, M., Wright, J. P., & Vaughn, M. G. (2009). Gene—Environment interplay and delinquent involvement evidence of direct, indirect, and interactive effects. *Journal of Adolescent Research, 24*(2), 147–168.

Beaver, K. M., Wright, J. P., DeLisi, M., Walsh, A., Vaughn, M. G., Boisvert, D., et al. (2007). A gene × gene interaction between DRD2 and DRD4 is associated with conduct disorder and antisocial behavior in males. *Behavioral and Brain Functions, 3*(1), 1.

Belsky, J., Conger, R., & Capaldi, D. M. (2009). The intergenerational transmission of parenting: Introduction to the special section. *Developmental Psychology, 45*(5), 1201.

Ben-David, V., Jonson-Reid, M., Drake, B., & Kohl, P. (2015). The association between childhood maltreatment experiences and the onset of maltreatment perpetration in young adulthood controlling for proximal and distal factors. *Child Abuse and Neglect, 46*, 132–141.

Berger, L. M. (2004). Income, family structure, and child maltreatment risk. *Children and Youth Services Review, 26*(8), 725–748.

Berlin, L. J., Appleyard, K., & Dodge, K. A. (2011). Intergenerational continuity in child maltreatment: Mediating mechanisms and implications for prevention. *Child Development, 82*(1), 162–176.

Berzenski, S. R., Yates, T. M., & Egeland, B. (2014). A multidimensional view of continuity in intergenerational transmission of child maltreatment. In *Handbook of child maltreatment* (pp. 115–129). Netherlands: Springer.

Brown, G. R., & Anderson, B. (1991). Psychiatric morbidity in adult inpatients with childhood histories of sexual and physical abuse. *American Journal of Psychiatry, 148*(1), 55–61.

Brown, J., Cohen, P., Johnson, J. G., & Salzinger, S. (1998). A longitudinal analysis of risk factors for child maltreatment: Findings of a 17-year prospective study of officially recorded and self-reported child abuse and neglect. *Child Abuse and Neglect, 22*(11), 1065–1078.

Caspi, A., McClay, J., Moffitt, T. E., Mill, J., Martin, J., Craig, I. W., et al. (2002). Role of genotype in the cycle of violence in maltreated children. *Science, 297*(5582), 851–854.

Chaffin, M., Kelleher, K., & Hollenberg, J. (1996). Onset of physical abuse and neglect: Psychiatric, substance abuse, and social risk factors from prospective community data. *Child Abuse and Neglect, 20*(3), 191–203.

Conger, R. D., Belsky, J., & Capaldi, D. M. (2009). The intergenerational transmission of parenting: closing comments for the special section. *Developmental Psychology, 45*(5), 1276.

Conger, R. D., Schofield, T. J., Neppl, T. K., & Merrick, M. T. (2013). Disrupting intergenerational continuity in harsh and abusive parenting: The importance of a nurturing relationship with a romantic partner. *Journal of Adolescent Health, 53*(4), S11–S17.

Cort, N. A., Toth, S. L., Cerulli, C., & Rogosch, F. (2011). Maternal intergenerational transmission of childhood multitype maltreatment. *Journal of Aggression, Maltreatment & Trauma, 20*(1), 20–39.

Coulton, C. J., Crampton, D. S., Irwin, M., Spilsbury, J. C., & Korbin, J. E. (2007). How neighborhoods influence child maltreatment: A review of the literature and alternative pathways. *Child Abuse and Neglect, 31*, 1117–1142.

DiLillo, D., & Damashek, A. (2003). Parenting characteristics of women reporting a history of childhood sexual abuse. *Child Maltreatment, 8*(4), 319–333.

DiLillo, D., Tremblay, G. C., & Peterson, L. (2000). Linking childhood sexual abuse and abusive parenting: The mediating role of maternal anger. *Child Abuse and Neglect, 24*(6), 767–779.

Dixon, L., Browne, K., & Hamilton-Giachritsis, C. (2005a). Risk factors of parents abused as children: a mediational analysis of the intergenerational continuity of child maltreatment (Part I). *Journal of Child Psychology and Psychiatry, 46*(1), 47–57.

Dixon, L., Browne, K., & Hamilton-Giachritsis, C. (2009). Patterns of risk and protective factors in the intergenerational cycle of maltreatment. *Journal of Family Violence, 24*(2), 111–122.

Dixon, L., Hamilton-Giachritsis, C., & Browne, K. (2005b). Attributions and behaviours of parents abused as children: A mediational analysis of the intergenerational continuity of child maltreatment (Part II). *Journal of Child Psychology and Psychiatry, 46*(1), 58–68.

Dong, M., Anda, R. F., Dube, S. R., Giles, W. H., & Felitti, V. J. (2003). The relationship of exposure to childhood sexual abuse to other forms of abuse, neglect, and household dysfunction during childhood. *Child Abuse and Neglect, 27*(6), 625–639.

Dong, M., Anda, R. F., Felitti, V. J., Dube, S. R., Williamson, D. F., Thompson, T. J., et al. (2004). The interrelatedness of multiple forms of childhood abuse, neglect, and household dysfunction. *Child Abuse and Neglect, 28*(7), 771–784.

Drake, B., & Pandey, S. (1996). Understanding the relationship between neighborhood poverty and specific types of child maltreatment. *Child Abuse and Neglect, 20*(11), 1003–1018.

Edwards, V. J., Holden, G. W., Felitti, V. J., & Anda, R. F. (2003). Relationship between multiple forms of childhood maltreatment and adult mental health in community respondents: results from the adverse childhood experiences study. *American Journal of Psychiatry, 160*(8), 1453–1460.

Ertem, I. O., Leventhal, J. M., & Dobbs, S. (2000). Intergenerational continuity of child physical abuse: How good is the evidence? *The Lancet, 356*(9232), 814–819.

Etter, D. J., & Rickert, V. I. (2013). The complex etiology and lasting consequences of child maltreatment. *Journal of Adolescent Health, 53*(4), S39–S41.

Felitti, V. J., Anda, R. F., Nordenberg, D., Williamson, D. F., Spitz, A. M., Edwards, V., Koss, M. P., & Marks, J. S. (1998). Relationship of childhood abuse and household dysfunction to many of the leading causes of death in adults: The Adverse Childhood Experiences (ACE) study. *American Journal of Preventive Medicine, 14*, 245–258.

Fergusson, D. M., Boden, J. M., & Horwood, L. J. (2008). Exposure to childhood sexual and physical abuse and adjustment in early adulthood. *Child Abuse and Neglect, 32*, 607–619.

Frias-Armenta, M. (2002). Long-term effects of child punishment on Mexican women: A structural model. *Child Abuse and Neglect, 26*(4), 371–386.

Geiger, J. M., & Schelbe, L. (2014). Stopping the cycle of abuse and neglect: A call to action to focus on pregnant and parenting foster youth. *Journal of Public Child Welfare, 8*, 25–50.

Geiger, J. M., Schelbe, L., Hayes, M. J., Kawam, E., Cary Katz, C., & Klika, J. B. (2015). Intergenerational transmission of maltreatment: Ending a family tradition. In D. Daro, A. C. Donnelly, L. A. Huang, & B. Powell (Eds.), *Advances in child abuse prevention knowledge*. New York: Springer.

Gilbert, R., Widom, C. S., Browne, K., Fergusson, D., Webb, E., & Janson, S. (2009). Burden and consequences of child maltreatment in high-income countries. *The Lancet, 37*, 68–81.

Guo, G., Roettger, M. E., & Shih, J. C. (2007). Contributions of the DAT1 and DRD2 genes to serious and violent delinquency among adolescents and young adults. *Human Genetics, 121*(1), 125–136.

Herrenkohl, T. I., Hong, S., Klika, J. B., Herrenkohl, R. C., & Russo, M. J. (2013). Developmental impacts of child abuse and neglect related to adult mental health, substance use, and physical health. *Journal of Family Violence, 28*(2), 191–199.

Herzberger, S. D. (1990). The cyclical pattern of child abuse: A study of research methodology. *The American Behavioral Scientist, 33*(5), 529.

Heyman, R. E., & Smith Slep, A. M. (2002). Do child abuse and interparental violence lead to adulthood family violence? *Journal of Marriage and Family, 64*(4), 864–870.
Hunter, R. S., & Kilstrom, N. (1979). Breaking the cycle in abusive families. *The American Journal of Psychiatry, 136*(10), 1320–1322.
Institute of Medicine & National Research Council. (2014). *New directions in child abuse and neglect research*. Washington, DC: The National Academies Press.
Jaffee, S. R., Bowes, L., Ouellet-Morin, I., Fisher, H. L., Moffitt, T. E., Merrick, M. T., et al. (2013). Safe, stable, nurturing relationships break the intergenerational cycle of abuse: A prospective nationally representative cohort of children in the United Kingdom. *Journal of Adolescent Health, 53*(4), S4–S10.
Jonson-Reid, M., Drake, B., & Kohl, P. L. (2009). Is the overrepresentation of the poor in child welfare caseloads due to bias or need? *Children and Youth Services Review, 31*(3), 422–427.
Jonson-Reid, M., Kohl, P. L., & Drake, B. (2012). Child and adult outcomes of chronic child maltreatment. *Pediatrics, 129*, 839–845.
Kaufman, J., & Zigler, E. (1987). Do abused children become abusive parents? *American Journal of Orthopsychiatry, 57*(2), 186.
Kim, K. (2012). The role of culture in theories of the intergenerational transmission of violence. *Child and Family Social Work, 17*, 395–405.
Kotch, J. B., Browne, D. C., Dufort, V., Winsor, J., & Catellier, D. (1999). Predicting child maltreatment in the first 4 years of life from characteristics assessed in the neonatal period. *Child Abuse and Neglect, 23*(4), 305–319.
Kunitz, S. J., Levy, J. E., McCloskey, J., & Gabriel, K. R. (1998). Alcohol dependence and domestic violence as sequelae of abuse and conduct disorder in childhood. *Child Abuse and Neglect, 22*(11), 1079–1091.
Leifer, M., Kilbane, T., Jacobsen, T., & Grossman, G. (2004). A three-generational study of transmission of risk for sexual abuse. *Journal of Clinical Child and Adolescent Psychology, 33*(4), 662–672.
Leve, L. D., Khurana, A., & Reich, E. B. (2015). Intergenerational transmission of maltreatment: A multilevel examination. *Development and Psychopathology, 27*, 1429–1442.
Locke, T. F., & Newcomb, M. D. (2003). Childhood maltreatment, parental alcohol/drug-related problems, and global parental dysfunction. *Professional Psychology: Research and Practice, 34*, 73–79.
Lounds, J. J., Borkowski, J. G., & Whitman, T. L. (2006). The potential for child neglect: The case of adolescent mothers and their children. *Child Maltreatment, 11*(3), 281–294.
MacMillan, H. L., Jamieson, E., Wathen, C. N., Boyle, M. H., Walsh, C. A., Omura, J., et al. (2007). Development of a policy-relevant child maltreatment research strategy. *Milbank Quarterly, 85*(2), 337–374.
McWey, L. M., Pazdera, A. L., Vennum, A., & Wojciak, A. S. (2013). Intergenerational patterns of maltreatment in families at risk for foster care. *Journal of Marital and Family Therapy, 39*(2), 133–147.
Merritt, D. H. (2009). Child abuse potential: Correlates with child maltreatment rates and structural measures of neighborhoods. *Children and Youth Services Review, 31*, 927–934.
Moffitt, T. E. (2005). The new look of behavioral genetics in developmental psychopathology: Gene-environment interplay in antisocial behaviors. *Psychological Bulletin, 131*(4), 533–554.
Moffitt, T. E., & Caspi, A. (2003). Preventing the intergenerational continuity of antisocial behaviour: Implications of partner violence. *Early Prevention of Adult Antisocial Behaviour* (pp. 109–129).
Neugebauer, R. (2000). Research on intergenerational transmission of violence: The next generation. *The Lancet, 355*(9210), 1116–1117.
Newcomb, M. D., & Locke, T. F. (2001). Intergenerational cycle of maltreatment: A popular concept obscured by methodological limitations. *Child Abuse and Neglect, 25*(9), 1219–1240.
Ogden, P., Minton, K., & Pain, C. (2006). *Trauma and the body: A sensorimotor approach to psychotherapy*. New York: W.W. Norton & Company.
Pears, K. C., & Capaldi, D. M. (2001). Intergenerational transmission of abuse: A two-generational prospective study of an at-risk sample. *Child Abuse and Neglect, 25*(11), 1439–1461.

Radey, M., Schelbe, L., McWey, L. M., Holtrop, K., & Canto, A. I. (2016). "It's really overwhelming": Parent and service provider perspectives of parents aging out of foster care. *Children and Youth Services Review, 67*, 1–10.

Renner, L., & Slack, K. S. (2006). Intimate partner violence and child maltreatment: Understanding intra- and intergenerational connections. *Child Abuse and Neglect, 30*(6), 599–617.

Schofield, T. J., Lee, R. D., & Merrick, M. T. (2013). Safe, stable, nurturing relationships as a moderator of intergenerational continuity of child maltreatment: A meta-analysis. *Journal of Adolescent Health, 53*(4), S32–S38.

Seltmann, L. A., & Wright, M. O. D. (2013). Perceived parenting competencies following childhood sexual abuse: A moderated mediation analysis. *Journal of Family Violence, 28*(6), 611–621.

Sidebotham, P., Golding, J., & ALSPAC Study Team. (2001). Child maltreatment in the "Children of the Nineties": A longitudinal study of parental risk factors. *Child Abuse & Neglect, 25*(9), 1177–1200.

Slack, K. S., Holl, J. L., McDaniel, M., Yoo, J., & Bolger, K. (2004). Understanding the risks of child neglect: An exploration of poverty and parenting characteristics. *Child Maltreatment, 9*(4), 395–408.

Smith, C. A., Ireland, T. O., Park, A., Elwyn, L., & Thornberry, T. P. (2011). Intergenerational continuities and discontinuities in intimate partner violence: A two-generation prospective study. *Journal of Interpersonal Violence, 26*, 3720–3752.

Straus, M. A. (1979). Family patterns and child abuse in a nationally representative American sample. *Child Abuse and Neglect, 3*(1), 213–225.

Thompson, R. (2006). Exploring the link between maternal history of childhood victimization and child risk of maltreatment. *Journal of Trauma Practice, 5*(2), 57–72.

Thornberry, T. P., & Henry, K. L. (2013). Intergenerational continuity in maltreatment. *Journal of Abnormal Child Psychology, 41*(4), 555–569.

Thornberry, T. P., Henry, K. L., Smith, C. A., Ireland, T. O., Greenman, S. J., & Lee, R. D. (2013). Breaking the cycle of maltreatment: The role of safe, stable, and nurturing relationships. *Journal of Adolescent Health, 53*(4), S25–S31.

Thornberry, T. P., Knight, K. E., & Lovegrove, P. J. (2012). Does maltreatment beget maltreatment? A systematic review of the intergenerational literature. *Trauma, Violence, & Abuse, 13*(3), 135–152.

Valentino, K., Nuttall, A., Comas, M., Borkowski, J., & Akai, C. (2012). Intergenerational continuity of child abuse among adolescent mothers: authoritarian parenting, community violence, and race. *Child Maltreatment, 17*, 172–181.

Widom, C. S. (1989). Does violence beget violence? A critical examination of the literature. *Psychological Bulletin, 106*(1), 3–28.

Widom, C. S. (1998). Child victims: Searching for opportunities to break the cycle of violence. *Applied and Preventive Psychology, 7*(4), 225–234.

Widom, C. S. (2015). Reflection: Intergenerational transmission of child maltreatment. In D. Daro, A. C. Donnelly, L. A. Huang, & B. J. Powell (Eds.), *Advances in child abuse prevention knowledge* (pp. 83–84). New York: Springer International Publishing.

Widom, C. S., & Brzustowicz, L. M. (2006). MAOA and the "cycle of violence:" Childhood abuse and neglect, MAOA genotype, and risk for violent and antisocial behavior. *Biological psychiatry, 60*(7), 684–689.

Widom, C. S., Czaja, S., & Dutton, M. A. (2014). Child abuse and neglect and intimate partner violence victimization and perpetration: A prospective investigation. *Child Abuse and Neglect, 38*(4), 650–663.

Widom, C. S., & Wilson, H. W. (2015). Intergenerational transmission of violence. In J. Lindert & I. Levav (Eds.), *Violence and mental health* (pp. 27–45). Netherlands: Springer.

Chapter 7
Prevention and Intervention Strategies to Address Intergenerational Transmission of Child Maltreatment

7.1 Incorporating Intergenerational Transmission of Child Maltreatment Knowledge into Intervention and Prevention Strategies

Why should the intergenerational transmission of child maltreatment (ITCM) be considered in intervention and prevention strategies since most parents who were abused as children do not abuse their children? The answer is fairly simple: because we currently do not fully understand the mechanisms of child maltreatment. While we know that the majority of children who are abused by their parents do not grow up and abuse their children, we know that some of them do (e.g., Kaufman and Zigler 1987; Pears and Capaldi 2001; Sidebotham et al. 2001; Widom and Wilson 2015). Experiencing maltreatment as a child does not sentence a parent's own children to a childhood of maltreatment. We cannot assume that parents who were abused as children will perpetrate child maltreatment. Yet we know that a parental history of maltreatment is one identified risk factor.

Intervention and prevention strategies can incorporate research that has identified risk factors. This has been done with other risk factors, for example, adolescent parenting. Programs have been developed specifically to address the needs of young parent and provide them with the skills and resources necessary to reduce the likelihood of future child maltreatment (Barth 2009). This same process can be done considering a parental history of child maltreatment and ITCM.

We are not suggesting that we think of child maltreatment deterministically. This could be potentially dangerous or detrimental. Herzberger (1990) recounts an incident where she and her colleague presented a paper criticizing the acceptance of ITCM as fact at a conference. Later, she received mail from parents who had been abused who said their presentation gave them hope because, despite having never abused their children, the parents lived in fear that one day they would harm their children since they had been abused as children. The letters expressed gratitude that they could overcome their past. Indeed, if parents who had been abused as children

L. Schelbe and J.M. Geiger, *Intergenerational Transmission of Child Maltreatment*, SpringerBriefs in Social Work,
DOI 10.1007/978-3-319-43824-5_7

believe that they are destined to abuse their children, is there not the potential for it to become a self-fulfilling prophecy? With the general acceptance of ITCM, why should someone who was abused as a child think any differently?

7.1.1 Prevention Approaches

We can look at intervention and prevention in a couple of ways. Knowing that there is not a 100 % transmission rate of children who were abused growing up and abusing their children, perhaps focusing on the survivors of child maltreatment for interventions and prevention strategies is misguided. But considering that we know ITCM is a possibility, knowing that parenting is challenging, and just because maltreatment is not occurring, does not mean that the parents are optimally parenting and may not need support and assistance. Therefore, targeting parents who were formerly abused as children does not seem that radical of a notion.

There are three types of prevention approaches: primary prevention, secondary prevention, and tertiary prevention. Primary prevention as it relates to child maltreatment includes an attempt to reduce the risks associated with child maltreatment before it occurs. This can include targeting groups of people who are more susceptible to child maltreatment (e.g., young children, young parents) and promoting protective factors. Primary prevention also includes enacting policies and programs that reduce the risks that are known to co-occur with child maltreatment. For example, the use of public service announcements that encourage positive parenting, family support and family strengthening programs, and parent education programs.

Secondary prevention involves reducing the impact of child maltreatment after it has occurred or when there is a known risk for future harm. This includes intervention to reduce child maltreatment from occurring again by addressing the risks associated with an incidence of child maltreatment and early intervention prior to harm. An example would be a parent who has left a young child unsupervised but no physical or emotional harm has occurred. Someone might intervene, recognizing a risk for harm and offer support or resources to reduce future harm or maltreatment. Examples of such programs include parenting education for a targeted group, home visiting programs for new mothers in their home, and respite care for families with children who have special needs.

Finally, tertiary prevention aims to minimize the impact of child maltreatment after it has occurred. For example, therapy, counseling, and a supportive environment after a child has experienced maltreatment can help the child manage the emotions following the experience of child maltreatment. Programs using a tertiary prevention approach include intensive family preservation services, parent mentor programs, and other mental health services.

Providing universal prevention and interventions is expensive. And currently, there is no widespread commitment to invest in prevention of child maltreatment despite repeated calls from experts that it would be cost-effective due to the high costs of child maltreatment. Therefore, from a purely economic perspective, it makes sense to have some targeted strategies to prevent child maltreatment. Since we know that ITCM is one risk factor, it makes sense to use the limited resources we have available for prevention and intervention to target those who may be likely to continue the cycle of violence. Another reason to consider targeted strategies to address child maltreatment is that interventions, broadly defined, may not be helpful to all people—especially some of those who need the interventions the most. Intervention and prevention strategies are not universally effective (Oxman et al. 1995); there is not a single approach that will work to prevent child maltreatment (Greeley 2009). As we will discuss later, ensuring strategies are tailored to address the unique needs of groups and populations versus "a one size fits all approach," which may be less effective (Widom 1998).

This chapter explores prevention and intervention strategies focused specifically on ITCM rather than looking at child maltreatment broadly. It is important to note that this is not an exhaustive list of child maltreatment prevention and intervention strategies. Rather, it is looking at how some of the specific and empirically supported child maltreatment prevention and intervention strategies can incorporate ITCM knowledge and potentially be adapted to meet specific groups' needs. It is important to note that to date there are no empirically supported programs specifically addressing ITCM according to the California Evidence-based Clearinghouse for Child Welfare (2016). This is not to say that parental history of maltreatment may not be addressed in interventions; it is only to emphasize that ITCM has not been the direct focus of interventions.

7.1.2 Guiding Principles

Nearly two decades ago, Widom (1998) described five principles to guide interventions focused on breaking the cycle of maltreated children becoming violent offenders in the future. While these principles are broadly addressing future violence and not just ITCM, their relevance to ITCM is great. The first principle is the earlier the intervention, the better. Second, child neglect needs to be addressed by interventions rather than by focusing entirely on physical and sexual abuse. The next principle is that "one size does not fit all" (Widom 1998, p. 230), and interventions need to be tailored to the specific needs and contexts. The fourth principle is a word of caution about surveillance, as some parents may be more likely to come into contact with mandated reporters. For example, those living in public housing and poverty may interact with social workers and law enforcement more frequently and therefore may be more likely to be reported for maltreatment. The final principle is that there is a need for people to have access to resources. In recent work, Widom and Wilson (2015) elaborate upon this,

> However, the children at greatest need often do not have access to these kinds of rigorous, evidence-based programs. Prevention programs that target the individual child alone are

> clearly not adequate. Early intervention programs that appear to be most effective have adopted a multidimensional approach with a variety of components, including family health care and parenting programs (p. 40).

Widom's (1998) principles remain relevant today in understanding interventions and prevention strategies of ITCM.

7.2 Empirically Supported Intervention and Prevention Strategies

There is a push to develop and adopt empirically supported interventions and preventions (Barth 2008; California Evidence-based Clearinghouse for Child Welfare 2016; Institute of Medicine and National Research Center 2014). As research on ITCM has expanded and knowledge has grown, scholars have discovered information that can be incorporated into prevention and intervention strategies. For example, the mediators and moderators in models looking at ITCM (e.g., social isolation, parental mental health) can be taken into consideration in efforts to reduce ITCM (Berlin et al. 2011). The information gained from ITCM research can be used to adapt empirically supported interventions and preventions.

Attempts should be made to reduce stigma in all intervention and prevention strategies. In the case of ITCM, just because a parent was maltreated as a child does not mean he or she is going to abuse his or her children. There is danger in stigmatizing parents at risk for perpetuating ITCM using the information to label parents as "potential abusers" (Sidebotham et al. 2001, p. 1196). Rather than labeling at-risk parents with negative labels, the goal should be to support parents as they negotiate how to raise their children.

7.2.1 Screening Tools

Identification of parents who are at risk for maltreating their children is important so that there can be targeted prevention and intervention efforts. A screening tool that takes into consideration risk factors including parental history of maltreatment is one idea (Dixon et al. 2005a; Newcomb and Locke 2001). However, caution should be taken with a screening tool as false positives are likely (Dixon et al. 2005a). Conversely, some parents who have not experienced maltreatment in childhood go on to develop high-risk profiles and maltreat their children (Dixon et al. 2009); if the screening tool overemphasizes parental history of maltreatment, these cases could be overlooked. Thus it is important that screening not be deterministic with using risk factors alone to make decisions; assessments should also include families' protective factors (Dixon et al. 2009).

A screening tool needs to take into consideration a wide range of factors as different risk factors are associated with different types of child maltreatment (Brown et al. 1998). The etiology of child maltreatment is complex and we cannot simply assume that parental history of child maltreatment is *the* deciding factor. Instead, we should attempt to tease out specific areas of need for the parent to maximize intervention impact and minimize wasting time and resources. For example, screening tools should be helpful in identifying what a parent needs, such as therapy, resources, housing assistance, or substance abuse treatment. Then, intervention should be focused on these areas versus providing too many services or programs that are too lengthy or complicated for families to engage in.

7.2.2 Home Visiting Programs

For prevention efforts, engaging parents in home visitation programs during pregnancy and early childhood has been found to reduce child maltreatment (Chaffin et al. 2012; Dodge et al. 2013; Lowell et al. 2011; Olds et al. 2007, 2010; Silovsky et al. 2011). There are multiple models of home visiting, which can involve either a trained professional or lay person visiting a family either prior to the birth of a child or afterward to provide support, information about parenting, and connections to available community resources. The number of visits varies as well as who is served. Some home visiting programs are universal while others target specific populations such as first time mothers in poverty. Scholars have recommended home visiting as a strategy specifically to address ITCM (Widom and Wilson 2015; Widom 1998).

7.2.3 Parent Training

Research suggests that risks of child maltreatment may be reduced through parent training that builds parenting skills and knowledge about child development (Barth and Haskins 2009; California Evidence-based Clearinghouse for Child Welfare 2016; Institute of Medicine and National Research Council 2014). Parent training programs that aim to reduce child maltreatment are often short-term, group-based interventions that utilize cognitive behavioral strategies and psychoeducation with parents. Research and evaluation of these programs is lacking, however, despite their widespread use with parents at risk for maltreatment.

There are empirically supported parenting intervention program that have been found to decrease the likelihood of future child maltreatment (Lundahl et al. 2006; Mikton and Butchart 2009). For example, The *Incredible Years*® is one of the most studied interventions (Webster-Stratton and Reid 2010). Other programs such as *Parent-Child Interaction Therapy (PCIT)*, *Nurturing Parenting Program*™, and *Triple P—Positive Parenting Practices*® aim to provide parents with simple and practical skills to manage children's behaviors and emotions, teach discipline techniques and nurturing behaviors, and build quality parent–child relationships. There are several promising models that also aim to preserve families including *Homebuilders®* and *Healthy Families®*. Both of these programs include a home-visiting component for at-risk families with young children. Both aim to promote child and family well-being, while preventing child maltreatment and removing the child from the home. Indeed, parenting education and training interventions have the potential to decrease child maltreatment as was demonstrated in a recent study of an evidence-based parenting intervention, the *Triple P—Positive Parenting Practices®* program. The program was found to decrease child maltreatment injuries and substantiated child maltreatment at a population level (Prinz et al. 2009). Several of these programs also include a community component to increase awareness about child maltreatment, highlight the need for more social support among parents, and mobilize community groups to promote improved outcomes (Daro and Dodge 2009). More research, however, is needed to understand parent training programs (Barth 2009; Mikton and Butchart 2009).

Prevention and intervention strategies that focus on improving parenting skills have been consistently recommended by those conducting ITCM research (Dixon et al. 2005b). Dixon and colleagues (2009) suggest that parent training be used, arguing "positive parenting programmes may be useful for all families presenting with a high risk profile regardless of parental childhood experiences, in order to enhance the quality of family life for both child(ren) and parents and reduce chances of maltreatment at a later stage in the child's life" (p. 120).

ITCM research findings have highlighted areas where parenting education may be effective. One area that parenting education can focus upon is consistent discipline, as research has found that a parental history of maltreatment, combined with poor discipline skills places parents at risk for continuing the cycle of maltreatment (Pears and Capaldi 2001). Interventions should address patterns, beliefs, and behaviors in parents who experienced maltreatment as children (McWey et al. 2013).

Parenting education as we have presented it thus far is focused on specific parents learning about parenting skills, however, it is also worthy to note the importance of public education and awareness as well as community prevention programs (see Institute of Medicine and National Research Council 2014). In addition to general messages about child abuse and neglect, information could be provided that history does not need to repeat itself and that the cycle of violence can be broken. Ensuring that people know ITCM which is not definitive and that people who experienced maltreatment as children can—and do—raise children safely and healthily may be helpful.

In addition, recent efforts include incorporating a trauma-informed approach to practice with children and families as well as promoting education and employment opportunities to minimize the co-occurring risks associated with child maltreatment and ITCM. By having knowledge and being cognizant of the risk and protective factors linked to ITCM, programs can target the needs of parents, children, and families that are not only tangible (e.g., cash benefits, housing, clothing, and food), but also in the way of social support, education, community, enrichment, and counseling. In order to prevent and reduce ITCM, service providers and other supports should intervene with families with a trauma-informed approach that addresses a parent's history of trauma and maltreatment as well.

7.2.4 Relationship Development

Relationships have the potential to decrease child maltreatment. In their meta-analysis of prospective three generation studies examining the impact of safe, stable, nurturing relationships on ITCM, Schofield and colleagues (2013) concluded that programs should use multiple components to target high-risk parents who had experienced child maltreatment and provide resources to improve parents' ability to develop and sustain healthy relationships with other adults. This conclusion speaks about how intervention and prevention efforts need to extend beyond simply focusing on developing parenting skills and must emphasize healthy relationships among couples/parents, parents and children, parents and other parents, and among children (see Chap. 5 for more information about relationships and support as a protective factor for child maltreatment and ITCM).

7.3 Addressing Culture

Throughout all child maltreatment prevention and intervention strategies, addressing culture is important (Institute of Medicine and National Resource Council 2014; Finno-Velasquez et al. 2015). Culture influences parenting practices and risk and protective factors that need to be taken into consideration with different groups of people (Lau 2006; Finno-Velasquez et al. 2015). There is a need to incorporate culture into the understanding of ITCM (Kim 2012) as there is evidence that there are important differences among racial and ethnic groups, and these differences should be taken into consideration in prevention and intervention strategies. For example, Valentino and colleagues (2012) found authoritarian parenting attitudes a protective factor for African American mothers and thus, concluded:

> Intervention programming should consider how to intervene against maltreatment without thwarting parenting practices that may be adaptive in particular cultural contexts…should the protective effects of authoritarian parenting attitudes among African American families continue to be supported with subsequent research, intervention programs may want to consider directly facilitating the development of these parenting attitudes among at-risk African American mothers while still reducing the use of physical punishment (p. 179).

It is important to note that culture extends beyond simple racial and ethnic differences and can include different identities and group membership such as the military, immigrant status, or lesbian, gay, bisexual, transgender, and queer (LGBTQ). Addressing culture and child maltreatment can occur at multiple levels:

the societal level, the program level, and the individual level (Finno-Velasquez et al. 2015). These levels need to be taken into consideration with ITCM prevention and intervention strategies.

7.4 Targeting Specific Populations

Knowing ITCM is a risk factor allows for targeted interventions. Various interventions have been developed to address the risks associated with child maltreatment and may be adapted to special populations and families affected by intergenerational maltreatment. Due to risk and protective factors, some populations may be more likely to experience ITCM. (see Chaps. 4 and 5 for information about risk and protective factors and ITCM.) Interventions can be designed to target specific at-risk groups of people and target specific risk factors. It is worth noting that research on prevention programs that simultaneously address a range of risk factors have not been rigorously evaluated (Barth 2009; Klevens and Whitaker 2007). Research has yet to determine conclusively if child maltreatment prevention programs must directly address risk factors (e.g., mental health problems, substance abuse, and intimate partner violence) or can solely address parenting practices (Barth 2009). However, there is a need to examine how risk factors of child maltreatment can be modified and child maltreatment prevented (Klevens and Whitaker 2007).

7.4.1 Child Welfare System Involved Families

Families involved in child welfare are a logical place to start as a target for prevention and intervention strategies attempting to address ITCM. Services provided to children and families after reunification and other permanency placements (e.g., adoption, guardianship) have the potential to decrease the number of children who reenter the child welfare system (Bellamy 2008). Efforts to reduce future maltreatment in families where there is documented maltreatment and concerns for child well-being is important, yet thinking about this solely as recidivism is shortsighted. We should be thinking of ensuring that intervention and prevention strategies are addressing the children who were maltreated to ensure that they do not grow up and abuse and neglect their children. Treatment should focus on the impact of trauma and maltreatment.

Targeting child welfare involved families likely will be complicated. Therefore, taking into consideration the various risk and protective factors is important. It cannot simply be focused on the single risk factor of parental history of maltreatment, but rather the myriad of other co-occurring factors related to maltreatment. The following example highlights this and the complexity of context including a lack of access to services. A study of second-generation child welfare involved families who all possessed a history of substance abuse found that such families had significantly more risk factors at time of case opening, and were two-thirds as likely to be reunified as first-generation child welfare involved families (Marshall et al. 2011). However, the effect of previous child welfare system involvement disappeared after the mental health diagnosis status was entered into the model; thus second-generation child welfare system involved caregivers had more mental health problems which was associated with a lower likelihood of reunification. The authors argue that this suggests the second-generation child welfare system involved caregivers who were not reunified experienced more mental health issues—which is also supported by previous research examining mental health outcomes in those who were maltreated as children and who entered the child welfare system (Marshall et al. 2011). The authors identify one explanation: it could be that services were not available and that court proceedings may be biased if parents' history of involvement in child protective services was known.

While targeting families involved with the child welfare system can be a strategy to reduce ITCM, it is also important to take into consideration potential surveillance or detection biases. In their 30-year prospective study of parents with a documented history of child maltreatment and a comparison group of parents without a documented history of child maltreatment, Widom and colleagues (2015) found that parents with a documented history of child maltreatment were 2.5 times more likely to have a report made to child protection services. Thus, they concluded that this suggests a detection or surveillance bias where there is the increased likelihood that child maltreatment will be reported.

Youth aging out of the child welfare system are a specific subgroup of those involved with the child welfare system who could be targeted for intervention and prevention strategies for ITCM. It is well documented that youth aging out are more likely than their peers who were not in foster care to become young parents (Dworsky and Courtney 2010; Oshima et al. 2013; Shpiegel and Cascardi 2015) and at risk for maltreating their children (Dworsky and DeCoursey 2009; Dworsky 2015). Before youth age out of the system, there is an opportunity to intervene and focus on developing parenting skills and other life skills that can decrease the chance of the cycle of violence being continued to another generation (Geiger and Schelbe 2014). Youth aging out who are already parenting may be a subgroup to target with interventions as recent research has highlighted that these parents desire to break the cycle of maltreatment and parent differently than they were parented (Aparicio et al. 2015, 2016; Radey et al. 2016).

7.4.2 *Families Affected by Intimate Partner Violence*

Research has found that children who were maltreated are more likely to experience intimate partner violence in their adult relationships (Kunitz et al. 1998; Smith et al. 2011; Stith et al. 2000). Likewise, the co-occurrence of child maltreatment and intimate partner violence is well documented along with its impact on ITCM

(Dixon et al. 2005b; Folsom et al. 2003; Renner and Slack 2006). A meta-analysis found that the rate of overlap between intimate partner violence and child maltreatment to be approximately 40 % (Appel and Holden 1998). Therefore, it is only logical to include targeting those experiencing or who have experienced intimate partner violence when considering child maltreatment prevention. However, there are few evaluations of programs that address intimate partner violence and child maltreatment (Barth 2009). Prevention efforts geared toward reducing ITCM should be sure to address intimate partner violence (Dixon et al. 2005b). Parents who either are experiencing or have experienced intimate partner violence may be dealing with victimization that impacts their ability to care for children and therefore interventions should take this into consideration (Renner and Slack 2006).

7.4.3 *Families and Parents Experiencing Trauma*

As a parents' history of maltreatment is only one risk factor for child maltreatment, interventions should take into consideration other commonly co-occurring risk factors such as recent experiences of violence and trauma (Thompson 2006). Children who experience maltreatment are at risk of living in a stressful environment and of being exposed to other events that can cause trauma including witnessing intimate partner violence, caregiver mental illness, caregiver substance abuse, and parental absence from the home (Dong et al. 2004; Felitti et al. 1998). As children who are maltreated—especially those where there is a history of ITCM—may live in stressful environments where trauma is present, it is necessary to take into consideration the full life span and understand the impact of trauma on development (Geiger et al. 2015).

The recognition of the importance of addressing trauma in child maltreatment intervention and prevention strategies is evident in the calls for trauma-informed care (Institute of Medicine and National Resource Council 2014). Thompson (2006) asserts, "Interventions that focus on these current aspects of formerly victimized adults' lives are likely to have far-reaching benefits not only for them, but for their children as well" (p. 70). For example, a parent who experiences trauma may be less responsive to their children's needs (Belsky et al. 2009).

7.4.4 *Parents Affected by Mental Health and Substance Abuse*

Parental mental health problems and substance abuse are risk factors for child maltreatment and ITCM. Research has found that parents with a history of child maltreatment who have mental health problems are more likely to maltreat their children compared to parents who have a history of maltreatment yet lack mental health problems (Berlin et al. 2011; Cort et al. 2011). Similarly, studies have found that substance abuse problems increase the risk of child maltreatment among parents who have experienced maltreatment themselves (Appleyard et al. 2011; Dixon et al. 2009; Jaffee et al. 2013; Kotch et al. 1999). More information on mental health and substance abuse as risk factors is in Chap. 4.

Despite the understanding of mental health and substance abuse as risk factors for child maltreatment, intervention and prevention programs rarely simultaneously focus on either mental health problems or substance abuse in addition to parenting skills (Barth 2009). While it may be worthy to develop such programs, focusing on parenting may have potential to assist with the other risk factors. Regardless of the approach, targeting parents with a history of child maltreatment, as well as a problem with mental health or substance abuse, has potential as a child maltreatment prevention strategy.

7.5 Recommendations for Evaluation of Intervention and Prevention Strategies

The importance of evaluating interventions and prevention strategies designed to reduce child maltreatment and ITCM cannot be overstated. There is a need to understand what works for whom and in what context. Prevention and intervention strategies should be adapted to meet the needs of different people. Child maltreatment is complicated. We need to make a concerted effort to figure out how we can prevent it and when it is not prevented, we must determine how we can make sure to reduce the detrimental effects of maltreatment and trauma and reduce ITCM.

It is important to remember that when addressing ITCM and child maltreatment, there is great diversity in the people who may benefit from interventions. Not all prevention strategies will work for all people. Evaluation of interventions and prevention efforts should take different populations into considerations. For example, some interventions and preventions may be tailored to meet the unique needs of youth aging out of the child welfare system who are parenting. Other strategies may specifically address the needs of parents who have experienced intimate partner violence.

To build a better understanding of how to reduce child maltreatment, more research on intervention and prevention is needed. Evaluations should be conducted on programs serving different groups of people. Interventions and prevention efforts should be examined in communities and within agencies (see Chap. 6 for more details about research and evaluation). The movement toward evidence-based practice is one that is also being applied to interventions involving children and families affected by child maltreatment and ITCM. Evidence-based practice (EBP) involves integrating the results of systematic research into social work practice by combining individual practitioners' experience with practices that have been subjected to rigorous testing and that addresses individual clients' needs and values (Gambrill 1999). EBP is a process that involves assessment, asking questions, searching for evidence, evaluating the evidence thoroughly, and taking action. Using EBP in our work with children and families affected by ITCM is important in ensuring that the interventions we use are ones that have been shown to work. Despite the benefits of using EBP and evidence-informed interventions, there are some limitations that have been noted. For example, EBP may not be generalizable to unique client populations on which they were not tested and the length of time it requires to adequately test an intervention or approach for it to qualify as EBP can limit its immediate utility.

7.6 Conclusion

Child maltreatment is an epidemic. It is important to develop effective prevention and intervention strategies. One risk factor is parental history of maltreatment. While not all children who are maltreated grow up to abuse and/or neglect their children, we know that some do. Thus incorporating ITCM prevention and intervention strategies is important. Some specific populations may be especially important to address in considering ITCM and prevention and interventions strategies, including: families involved with the child welfare system, families where intimate partner violence is present, and families where parents have experienced trauma.

References

Aparicio, E., Pecukonis, E. V., & O'Neale, S. (2015). "The love that I was missing": Exploring the lived experience of motherhood among teen mothers in foster care. *Children and Youth Services Review, 51*, 44–54.

Aparicio, E. M., Gioia, D., & Pecukonis, E. V. (2016). "I Can Get Through This and I Will Get Through This": The unfolding journey of teenage motherhood in and beyond foster care. *Qualitative Social Work.*

Appel, A. E., & Holden, G. W. (1998). The co-occurrence of spouse and physical child abuse: A review and appraisal. *Journal of Family Psychology, 12*(4), 578.

Appleyard, K., Berlin, L. J., Rosanbalm, K. D., & Dodge, K. A. (2011). Preventing early child maltreatment: Implications from a longitudinal study of maternal abuse history, substance use problems, and offspring victimization. *Prevention Science, 12,* 139e49.

Barth, R. P. (2008). The move to evidence-based practice: How well does it fit child welfare services? *Journal of Public Child Welfare, 2*(2), 145–171.

Barth, R. P. (2009). Preventing child abuse and neglect with parent training: Evidence and opportunities. *The Future of Children, 19*, 95–118.

Barth, R. P., & Haskins, R. (2009). Will parent training reduce abuse, enhance development, and save money? Let's find out. Future of Children Policy Brief. Retrieved from http://www.futureofchildren.org/futureofchildren/publications/docs/19_02_PolicyBrief_2.pdf

Bellamy, J. L. (2008). Behavioral problems following reunification of children in long-term foster care. *Children and Youth Services Review, 30*, 216–228.

Belsky, J., Conger, R., & Capaldi, D. M. (2009). The intergenerational transmission of parenting: Introduction to the special section. *Developmental Psychology, 45*(5), 1201.

Berlin, L. J., Appleyard, K., & Dodge, K. A. (2011). Intergenerational continuity in child maltreatment: Mediating mechanisms and implications for prevention. *Child Development, 82*(1), 162–176.

Brown, J., Cohen, P., Johnson, J. G., & Salzinger, S. (1998). A longitudinal analysis of risk factors for child maltreatment: Findings of a 17-year prospective study of officially recorded and self-reported child abuse and neglect. *Child Abuse and Neglect, 22*(11), 1065–1078.

California Evidence-based Clearinghouse for Child Welfare. (2016). *Program registry*. Retrieved from http://www.cebc4cw.org/home

Chaffin, M., Hecht, D., Bard, D., Silovsky, J. F., & Beasley, W. H. (2012). A statewide trial of the SafeCare home-based services model with parents in child protective services. *Pediatrics, 129*(3), 509–515.

Cort, N. A., Toth, S. L., Cerulli, C., & Rogosch, F. (2011). Maternal intergenerational transmission of childhood multitype maltreatment. *Journal of Aggression, Maltreatment & Trauma, 20*(1), 20–39.

Daro, D., & Dodge, K. A. (2009). Creating community responsibility for child protection: Possibilities and challenges. *The Future of Children, 19*(2), 67.

Dixon, L., Browne, K., & Hamilton-Giachritsis, C. (2005a). Risk factors of parents abused as children: a mediational analysis of the intergenerational continuity of child maltreatment (Part I). *Journal of Child Psychology and Psychiatry, 46*(1), 47–57.

Dixon, L., Browne, K., & Hamilton-Giachritsis, C. (2009). Patterns of risk and protective factors in the intergenerational cycle of maltreatment. *Journal of Family Violence, 24*(2), 111–122.

Dixon, L., Hamilton-Giachritsis, C., & Browne, K. (2005b). Attributions and behaviours of parents abused as children: A mediational analysis of the intergenerational continuity of child maltreatment (Part II). *Journal of Child Psychology and Psychiatry, 46*(1), 58–68.

Dodge, K. A., Goodman, W. B., Murphy, R., O'Donnell, K., & Sato, J. (2013). Toward population impact from home visiting. *Zero to Three, 33*(3), 17.

Dong, M., Anda, R. F., Felitti, V. J., Dube, S. R., Williamson, D. F., Thompson, T. J., et al. (2004). The interrelatedness of multiple forms of childhood abuse, neglect, and household dysfunction. *Child Abuse and Neglect, 28*(7), 771–784.

Dworsky, A. (2015). Child welfare services involvement among the children of young parents in foster care. *Child Abuse and Neglect, 45*, 68–79.

Dworsky, A., & Courtney, M. E. (2010). The risk of teenage pregnancy among transitioning foster youth: Implications for extending state care beyond age 18. *Children and Youth Services Review, 32*, 1351–1356.

Dworsky, A., & DeCoursey, J. (2009). *Pregnant and parenting foster youth: Their needs, their experiences*. Chicago: Chapin Hall Center for Children at the University of Chicago. Retrieved from http://www.chapinhall.org/sites/default/files/Pregnant_Foster_Youth_final_081109.pdf

Felitti, V. J., Anda, R. F., Nordenberg, D., Williamson, D. F., Spitz, A. M., Edwards, V., et al. (1998). Relationship of childhood abuse and household dysfunction to many of the leading causes of death in adults: The adverse childhood experiences (ACE) study. *American Journal of Preventive Medicine, 14*(4), 245–258.

Finno-Velasquez, M., Shuey, E. A., Kotake, C., & Miller, J. J. (2015). Cultural considerations in refining intervention designs. In D. Daro, A. C. Donnelly, L. A. Huang, & B. J. Powell (Eds.), *Advances in child abuse prevention knowledge* (pp. 93–117). New York: Springer International Publishing

Folsom, W. S., Christensen, M. L., Avery, L., & Moore, C. (2003). The co-occurrence of child abuse and domestic violence: An issue of service delivery for social service professionals. *Child and Adolescent Social Work Journal, 20*(5), 375–387.

Gambrill, E. (1999). Evidence based practice: An alternative to authority-based practice. *Families in Society, 80*(4), 341–350.

Geiger, J. M., & Schelbe, L. A. (2014). Stopping the cycle of child abuse and neglect: A call to action to focus on pregnant and parenting youth in and aging out of the foster care system. *Journal of Public Child Welfare, 8*, 25–50.

Geiger, J. M., Schelbe, L., Hayes, M. J., Kawam, E., Cary Katz, C., & Klika, J. B. (2015). Intergenerational transmission of maltreatment: Ending a family tradition. In D. Daro, A. C. Donnelly, L. A. Huang, & B. Powell (Eds.), *Advances in child abuse prevention knowledge*. New York: Springer.

Greeley, C. S. (2009). The future of child maltreatment prevention. *Pediatrics, 123*(3), 904–905.

Healthy Families America®. (2016). Retrieved from http://www.healthyfamiliesamerica.org

Herzberger, S. D. (1990). The cyclical pattern of child abuse: A study of research methodology. *The American Behavioral Scientist, 33*(5), 529.

Incredible Years®. (2016). Retrieved from http://incredibleyears.com/

Institute for Family Development. (2016). Homebuilders®: Intensive family preservation service and intensive family reunification services. Retrieved from http://www.institutefamily.org/programs_ifps.asp

Institute of Medicine & National Research Council. (2014). *New directions in child abuse and neglect research*. Washington, DC: The National Academies Press.

Jaffee, S. R., Bowes, L., Ouellet-Morin, I., Fisher, H. L., Moffitt, T. E., Merrick, M. T., et al. (2013). Safe, stable, nurturing relationships break the intergenerational cycle of abuse: A prospective nationally representative cohort of children in the United Kingdom. *Journal of Adolescent Health, 53*(4), S4–S10.

Kaufman, J., & Zigler, E. (1987). Do abused children become abusive parents? *American Journal of Orthopsychiatry, 57*(2), 186.

Kim, K. (2012). The role of culture in theories of the intergenerational transmission of violence. *Child and Family Social Work, 17*(4), 395–405.

Klevens, J., & Whitaker, D. J. (2007). Primary prevention of child physical abuse and neglect: Gaps and promising directions. *Child Maltreatment, 12*(4), 364–377.

Kotch, J. B., Browne, D. C., Dufort, V., Winsor, J., & Catellier, D. (1999). Predicting child maltreatment in the first 4 years of life from characteristics assessed in the neonatal period. *Child Abuse and Neglect, 23*(4), 305–319.

Kunitz, S. J., Levy, J. E., McCloskey, J., & Gabriel, K. R. (1998). Alcohol dependence and domestic violence as sequelae of abuse and conduct disorder in childhood. *Child Abuse and Neglect, 22*(11), 1079–1091.

Lau, A. S. (2006). Making the case for selective and directed cultural adaptations of evidence-based treatments: examples from parent training. *Clinical Psychology: Science and Practice, 13*(4), 295–310.

Lowell, D. I., Carter, A. S., Godoy, L., Paulicin, B., & Briggs-Gowan, M. J. (2011). A randomized controlled trial of Child FIRST: A comprehensive home-based intervention translating research into early childhood practice. *Child Development, 82*(1), 193–208.

Lundahl, B. W., Nimer, J., & Parsons, B. (2006). Preventing child abuse: A meta-analysis of parent training programs. *Research on Social Work Practice, 16*(3), 251–262.

Marshall, J. M., Huang, H., & Ryan, J. P. (2011). Intergenerational families in child welfare: Assessing needs and estimating permanency. *Children and Youth Services Review, 33*(6), 1024–1030.

McWey, L. M., Pazdera, A. L., Vennum, A., & Wojciak, A. S. (2013). Intergenerational patterns of maltreatment in families at risk for foster care. *Journal of Marital and Family Therapy, 39*(2), 133–147.

Mikton, C., & Butchart, A. (2009). Child maltreatment prevention: A systematic review of reviews. *Bulletin of the World Health Organization, 87*(5), 353–361.

Newcomb, M. D., & Locke, T. F. (2001). Intergenerational cycle of maltreatment: A popular concept obscured by methodological limitations. *Child Abuse and Neglect, 25*(9), 1219–1240.

Nurturing Parenting Program. (2016). Retrieved from http://www.nurturingparenting.com/

Olds, D. L., Kitzman, H. J., Cole, R. E., Hanks, C. A., Arcoleo, K. J., Anson, E. A., et al. (2010). Enduring effects of prenatal and infancy home visiting by nurses on maternal life course and government spending: Follow-up of a randomized trial among children at age 12 years. *Archives of Pediatrics and Adolescent Medicine, 164*(5), 419–424.

Olds, D. L., Sadler, L., & Kitzman, H. (2007). Programs for parents of infants and toddlers: Recent evidence from randomized trials. *Journal of Child Psychology and Psychiatry, 48*(3–4), 355–391.

Oshima, K. M. M., Narendorf, S. C., & McMillen, J. C. (2013). Pregnancy risk among older youth transitioning out of foster care. *Children and Youth Services Review, 35*(10), 1760–1765.

Oxman, A. D., Thomson, M. A., Davis, D. A., & Haynes, B. (1995). No magic bullets: A systematic review of 102 trials of interventions to improve professional practice. *Canadian Medical Association Journal, 153*(10), 1424–1431.

Parent-Child Interaction Therapy. (2016). Retrieved from http://www.pcit.org/

Pears, K. C., & Capaldi, D. M. (2001). Intergenerational transmission of abuse: A two-generational prospective study of an at-risk sample. *Child Abuse and Neglect, 25*(11), 1439–1461.

Prinz, R. J., Sanders, M. R., Shapiro, C. J., Whitaker, D. J., & Lutzker, J. R. (2009). Population-based prevention of child maltreatment: The US Triple P system population trial. *Prevention Science, 10*(1), 1–12.

Radey, M., Schelbe, L., McWey, L. M., Holtrop, K., & Canto, A. I. (2016). "It's really overwhelming": Parent and service provider perspectives of parents aging out of foster care. *Children and Youth Services Review, 67*, 1–10.

Renner, L., & Slack, K. S. (2006). Intimate partner violence and child maltreatment: Understanding intra- and intergenerational connections. *Child Abuse and Neglect, 30*(6), 599–617.

Schofield, T. J., Lee, R. D., & Merrick, M. T. (2013). Safe, stable, nurturing relationships as a moderator of intergenerational continuity of child maltreatment: A meta-analysis. *Journal of Adolescent Health, 53*(4), S32–S38.

Shpiegel, S., & Cascardi, M. (2015). Adolescent parents in the first wave of the national youth in transition database. *Journal of Public Child Welfare, 9*(3), 277–298.

Sidebotham, P., Golding, J., & ALSPAC Study Team. (2001). Child maltreatment in the "Children of the Nineties": A longitudinal study of parental risk factors. *Child Abuse & Neglect, 25*(9), 1177–1200.

Silovsky, J. F., Bard, D., Chaffin, M., Hecht, D., Burris, L., Owora, A., et al. (2011). Prevention of child maltreatment in high-risk rural families: A randomized clinical trial with child welfare outcomes. *Children and Youth Services Review, 33*(8), 1435–1444.

Smith, C. A., Ireland, T. O., Park, A., Elwyn, L., & Thornberry, T. P. (2011). Intergenerational continuities and discontinuities in intimate partner violence: A two-generation prospective study. *Journal of Interpersonal Violence, 26*, 3720–3752.

Stith, S. M., Rosen, K. H., Middleton, K. A., Busch, A. L., Lundeberg, K., & Carlton, R. P. (2000). The intergenerational transmission of spouse abuse: A meta-analysis. *Journal of Marriage and Family, 62*(3), 640–654.

Thompson, R. (2006). Exploring the link between maternal history of childhood victimization and child risk of maltreatment. *Journal of Trauma Practice, 5*(2), 57–72.

Triple P—Positive Parenting Program®. (2016). Retrieved from http://www.triplep.net/glo-en/home/

Valentino, K., Nuttall, A., Comas, M., Borkowski, J., & Akai, C. (2012). Intergenerational continuity of child abuse among adolescent mothers: authoritarian parenting, community violence, and race. *Child Maltreatment, 17*, 172–181.

Webster-Stratton, C., & Reid, M. J. (2010). Adapting the Incredible years, an evidence-based parenting programme, for families involved in the child welfare system. *Journal of Children's Services, 5*(1), 25–42.

Widom, C. S. (1998). Child victims: Searching for opportunities to break the cycle of violence. *Applied and Preventive Psychology, 7*(4), 225–234.

Widom, C. S., Czaja, S. J., & DuMont, K. A. (2015). Intergenerational transmission of child abuse and neglect: Real or detection bias? *Science, 347*(6229), 1480–1485.

Widom, C. S., & Wilson, H. W. (2015). Intergenerational transmission of violence. In J. Lindert & I. Levav (Eds.), *Violence and mental health* (pp. 27–45). Netherlands: Springer.

FSC
www.fsc.org
MIX
Papier | Fördert
gute Waldnutzung
FSC® C083411

Kolibri 360 GmbH
Ferdinand-Jühlke-Straße 7
99095 Erfurt, Deutschland
produktsicherheit@kolibri360.de